THINK
AND
GROW
VEGAN

THINK AND GROW VEGAN

Glen John Jones

Gradually adopt a plant-based diet
with confidence in five stages

**FIRST
NEVER
SECOND**

First published in the United Kingdom in 2019 by
First Never Second, www.firstneversecond.com

Think and Grow Vegan - ©2019 Glen John Jones

1 2 3 4 5 6 7 / 22 21 20 19

Written by Glen John Jones
Copyediting by Ameesha Smith-Green
Design by Radim Malinic

British Library Cataloguing-in-Publication Data.
A catalogue record for this book is available from the British Library

ISBN 978-1-9161188-0-5

Printed and bound in Great Britain by Clays Ltd, Elcograf S.p.A

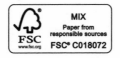

CONTENTS

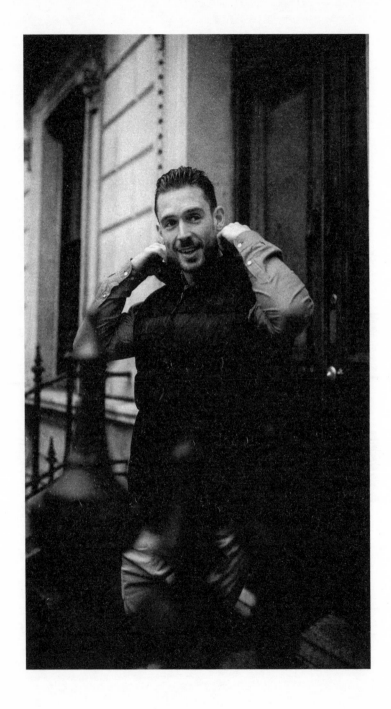

About the Author

Glen John Jones is a Personal Trainer and Deep Tissue Masseuse based in South London. Having been involved in the fitness industry since 2008, he's helped many people work towards and reach their goals. His tenure in the industry includes working with the most well-known commercial gyms and sports supplement companies in the UK, plus a cheeky stint "down under" in Australia!

Glen strives for and works with a wide range of clients—each with different personalities, body types, and goals. His clientele varies from those who are relatively new to training but want to lose weight and tone up ... to the all-round, fit, gym-goer who wants to take things up a notch ... to the competitive Ironman looking to qualify for the World Championships in a few years' time. His prerogative for all of his clients is to give them more energy and zing in every part of their day.

A firm believer that there isn't a "one size fits all approach" to achieving fitness goals, Glen takes a multidimensional approach to training with close attention to detail. This can include many specific protocols benefiting strength, mobility, core, endurance, sports conditioning, corrective exercise, injury rehabilitation, body composition, plant-based nutrition, and overall energy levels.

In 2016, Glen was approached by an old friend from nursery who had gained investment to open a boutique fitness studio in the local area. They became business partners, opening Studio 234. These old school pals were featured in the local Guardian on page 3: #Lifegoals. Glen now does the majority of his personal training and massage therapy at Studio 234.

In 2017, Glen competed in the Reebok Spartan Beast in Edinburgh, Scotland, coming second out of around 800 participants. This subsequently led to him being featured on the BBC Good Food website as "The Vegan Personal Trainer", where Glen explains how his diet affects his career and his clients.

Despite this book tip-toeing into certain aspects of nutrition and the value of meal preparation, Glen is admittedly not a big lover of cooking, being neither particularly good at it, nor naturally passionate about it. For this reason, he truly believes that if he can adopt a plant-based diet without too much drama and feel better all over for this, then anyone can! Glen's story is relatable to many who lead busy lifestyles and want to feel better.

When not training his clients, Glen enjoys swimming, cycling, running, indoor bouldering, hiking and training at Studio 234 in all things fitness. If he is due to compete in an upcoming event, his training regime becomes more intense and specific to the task at hand and this ultimately shapes his routine, including his nutrition.

His future projects to include more books, delving into other specific subjects such as fitness, and online training and nutrition programmes for clients worldwide.

You can find Glen at:
Instagram: @glenjohnjones
Website: glenjohnjones.com

Instagram: @thinkandgrowvegan
Website: thinkandgrowvegan.com

Why I wrote this book

"I want to become a vegan, but I don't know how to". I truly realised the sense of urgency to write this book based on the sheer amount of times people said this to me, and what's more, so many different types of people. After brief conversations when "the vegan topic" arose, sometimes people would come back to me and ask how I did it. Sometimes, the outcome was that they'd want to try it themselves— or at least eat less meat. Some people even told me that I should write a book ... so here we are!

Come the final stage of my own plant-based journey, receiving criticism and compliments had become the norm, albeit it was a bit weird that so many people wanted to discuss my diet! I could only take the fact that people were talking to me openly about how they wanted to adopt a plant-based diet for themselves as a compliment. At least I was inspiring them and not putting them off, I thought. Seeing as most people think all vegans are annoying and on the verge of malnutrition, people seemed pleasantly surprised by my mannerisms not changing for the worse following my change in diet.

Naturally, many people have apprehensions and reasons for not transitioning to a plant-based diet—even if they want to. From misconceptions to social stigmas all the way to failed trials of the mainstream vegan diet suggested in society. The combination of social stigmas, misconceptions, and failed vegan diet attempts arguably puts people off going beyond even thinking about becoming vegan. Let alone trying it out.

However, what I found is that when people saw me doing well at the plant-based diet, then they realised that it's possible for them too. This is what led to Think and Grow Vegan, the need for a better way to switch to a plant-based diet. From experience, you "grow" into the vegan thing, so it fits you.

If you're not a fan of the word "vegan" right now, don't worry! It means the same as "plant-based diet", and I use the two interchangeably in this book. The same goes for a "normal", mainstream, meat-eater diet, AKA a conventional/traditional/ convenient Western diet.

Although potentially controversial and off-putting, I've used the word "vegan" based on the sheer reality that if you adopt a plant-based diet, then you and your food would technically be known by the title of "vegan" in society. However, the further you go on your personal journey, it's likely that you'll care less about how you describe your diet.

Although the word "vegan" has some negative connotations in today's society, I truly believe that the 'V' word will one day be the norm, describing people who eat a plant-based diet. For now, know that "vegan" is literally just a name. A name that means as much or as little as you want it to mean.

I delayed my own transition to becoming a vegan for months before even mentioning to a friend that I was "loosely considering looking into it". He'd been on the vegan vibes for years, so I wanted to pick his brain before going any further. When I initially approached him with "I'd like to know more about the diet/lifestyle/general vegan stuff", he literally burst out laughing! "Vegan?!...You?!" he said.

At the time, I couldn't have been any further opposite. I used to eat beef and eggs for breakfast and carry cooked chicken thighs around with me in Tupperware for lunch! Once he could contain himself, he said, "Come back to me in a few months and if you're still interested, and we'll have a sit down." It was only after that when I really started to believe that it could be done, when we explored the ins and outs of it. This book is the upshot.

Who this book is for

Coming from my background in the fitness industry as a Personal Trainer, I know that people's mindsets can become a bit "stall-ish" when it comes to making a change, even if it's for the better. They wait for the perfect time, instead of making it the perfect time.

Many people have approached me for personal training in the past, but they change their mind before we've even begun. If only I had a pound for every time someone said to me: "I just want to get a bit fitter first..." They want to get fit BEFORE they get fit. Makes no sense, right? As the old saying goes: "Strike while the iron is hot". So if and when you have the desire to change to a plant-based diet—fucking go for it! Don't wait for the perfect time, because there's never a perfect time.

If you don't want to do it, then don't. I haven't written this book for people who don't want to make the transition, or for people who are on the fence about it. I believe that being vegan is not something you should have to convince someone to do. They should want to do it. Eating meat and animal products isn't exactly illegal, is it?! I'm not trying to coerce anyone into doing something they're not sure of. Similarly, I wouldn't work with a client who wasn't sure about training with me. I've written this book for the people who WANT to do it.

So, when the time comes and you've made the decision to crack on, this book will give you some anecdotes to take away with you, and get you up to speed on the subjects that surround the plant-based diet. No pressure.

Likewise, there are many reasons why you might want to adopt a plant-based diet, from environmental ones to economic, ethical to health, among other things. This book isn't just for those who are doing it for health reasons, ethical reasons, or anything else. It's for anyone who wants to take up a plant-based diet for whatever reason fits them and their lifestyle.

What this book is about

Put simply, this book is about how to think and grow vegan. As a diet choice, veganism is growing in take-up, but there's still a lack of realistic, good advice out there on how to make a healthy, comfortable transition. This book shows you some ideas on how you could make the transition to a plant-based diet smoother.

Let's look at the big picture of veganism in the UK:

- There is reportedly over 65 million people in the UK, and in 2016, 542,000 of those are said to identify as vegans. That's under 1% of the population, or less than 1 in 100.
- It's reported that almost half of all vegans are in the 15-34 age category (42%), compared to just 14% who are over 65.
- Geographically, 88% of vegans in the UK live in urban or suburban areas, compared to 12% in rural areas. Around 22% of all vegans in the UK live in London, more than any other region.
- As of 2016, almost twice as many vegans identify as female (63%) than male (37%).

With these stats in mind, there's a chance that you might not have talked to a vegan before, and don't know what it's like to transition to a plant-based diet in today's society. In this book, I'll let you in on what it's really like.

Let's get this straight from the start: I'm not the perfect vegan. In fact, there is no such thing. I certainly don't have the perfect diet. I'm not an environmentalist, economist, animal rights activist, or cardiologist. My knowledge of these topics is slight compared to the experts in these fields. As such, I don't go too deep in this book, and I didn't want to turn it into a science degree!

I'm the first person to admit that you can get much better insights into these topics if you go straight to the source, but it can also be pretty boring, so I've given you the headlines and key info here. My research comes from a diverse mix of mainstream publications, surveys, medical reports, studies, and popular beliefs gathered from experience. If you're interested, I provide references on the Think and Grow Vegan website, so you can look into these topics further. **Thinkandgrowvegan.com**

In the fitness industry, my role is to get clients from A to B (their goals), through all the ups and downs. Having done this for around a decade, I've developed a knack at getting the best out of people when they are dead serious about committing to change. I reverse-engineer the end result, then connect the dots (the how) for them along the way as they balance their work, family, social life, and the unexpected variables of life around their goals. I always do this with the utmost integrity and try to make it as jovial as possible for them while they push to greater heights. The same goes for this book.

I'll give you my honest personal account—shedding light on what it feels like to go through the gradual transition from meat eater to vegan in the modern world. I have lived and breathed all the thrills and spills of this for myself!

My story is the guide.

Life is what your goals are

You've no doubt heard the old saying: "Life is what you make it". To an extent, it is true. That being said, I personally believe that life is more about what your goals are than anything else.

Your whole life can change when you change your goals. However, to achieve new goals, you also have to change your life. This goes for your habits, mindset, training, nutrition, the people you hang around with, literally everything you're surrounded by.

To a degree, everything changes when you set and then act on a goal. Say you decide that you're going to work towards a plant-based diet, whether you realise it or not, that right there is a goal. From that point on, your life will change. All because you set that one goal. It's a life-changing decision.

A long-term goal will change more things over time than a short-term goal. This is because a long-term goal usually requires a greater magnitude of attention over an extended period of time. Especially if it's a massive goal! Define "massive goal": something that's going to be fucking difficult to achieve! Adhering to a plant-based diet can feel like this to some.

Due to the magnitude of what's required to reach a massive, long-term goal, it can be daunting for some, yet exciting for others. Either way, you'll feel less overwhelmed when you break a large goal down into a series of smaller stages. All of which take you closer to the big boy you really want in the end.

Going the "completely abolish" route to this diet works for some people. I personally went for the gradual route and have nothing but good things to say about the experience. What's more, I've been able to stick to it in nearly all situations, which is ultimately why I recommend doing it this way if you are indeed looking to make the transition.

How to read this book

You'll find that this book is laid out in five stages to reflect my gradual transition from a 'normal' meat-eater diet to a plant-based diet:

Stage One: Reduce.
Stage Two: Pescatarian.
Stage Three: Vegetarian.
Stage Four: Mostly Vegan.
Stage Five: Vegan.

In each of the five stages, there are three sub-sections:

Storytime
The thrills and spills. Exactly as it happened. Including some relevant citations where relevant. The backbone of the book.

Misconceptions
A subject relating to the story—usually a common belief in society about why a plant-based diet is a load of old toshwollop and is impossible to achieve. Sometimes, these misconceptions are inconclusive and require you to decide what you believe from my input and the evidence from both sides.

Summary
Found at the very end of each stage. Offers take-home tips. Literally wrapping up what we discussed in the storytime and misconceptions.

When reading this book, you can literally read the book from start to finish, or you can randomly open the book on any page, say when you're sitting on the toilet, and it will still flow! As such, you'll find that for every storytime, there is a misconception right after it. To help you distinguish between the subsections and stages, I've labelled the top of each page so you know exactly where you're at.

You might clock that the number of chapters varies at each stage. This emphasises the fact that your transition isn't a robotic system, a simple plan that anybody can follow to magically become a vegan in 12 weeks with a certificate at the end. A "one size fits all approach" doesn't cut it in the long term.

You have to get your hands dirty and find out what works for you...naturally! You have to be patient with it, learn from your mistakes, and understand that everyone's different. Sure, I'll offer lots of insights based on my own experience and provide evidence that takes everything into account. But ultimately, if you really want it to work for you, you'll find a way amongst your own priorities.

So if you're ready, let's crack on...

Stage One
REDUCE

I couldn't eat bacon anymore!

It was just another Tuesday evening, and my busiest day of the week had left me sprawled out on the sofa, belly up, exhausted. I tried to unwind from a full day of coaching. Typically, unwinding would be going for a walk or chatting on the phone with a friend. But this particular night, I was only mentally up for scrolling through social media instead. Thumbs at the ready, I flicked between Facebook, Instagram, and Youtube. I was looking for something funny or a useful snippet of information to indulge in, but I didn't find either. I did feel more rested though, so I went upstairs to brush my teeth.

About halfway up the stairs still looking at my phone, a video popped up on my Facebook feed. Unlike all the other videos I had scrolled past, it got my attention. So much so that stopped walking up the stairs. The video showed a sick piglet being held over a young girl's shoulder, and she was singing a lullaby to it. The piglet was crying, and you could see in its eyes how sad it was. The girl was also crying. The whole scenario reminded me of a mother and a baby. I had no idea why it got my attention and why I was so engrossed in that I watched it twice, but I took it as a sign.

The weird thing was, a couple of weeks before the video popped up, I was eating eggs, bacon, and spinach, and I couldn't finish the bacon. It was the first time in my life that I'd left any type of food uneaten on my plate. At the time, it was a regular, favourite breakfast of mine, but my brain got the better of my taste buds.

Another time, I was eating the very same breakfast when I had a flashback of watching a TV programme about tattooing. Bizarrely, I had seen the show around 10 years before, and rarely (if ever) watched TV anymore. I specifically remember the trainees were using pig flesh to practice their drawings on, as they said: "A pig's skin is the closest thing to human's skin." The flashback freaked me out so much that I spat the food out and felt rather sick.

Admittedly, it wasn't just bacon I was having this "problem" with—it was all pork or pork-based products. So ham, ham sandwiches, gammon, pork scratchings, bacon-flavoured crisps, pork pies, scotch eggs, you name it—I wasn't going near any of them anymore! Not that I ate them often anyway, as let's face it, they aren't the most healthy foods. But just the sight or thought of these foods brought back memories of that line from the tattoo show.

I tried eating bacon a few more times after that occasion, because I thought it was just me being stupid and that eating bacon was "normal". But the same thing happened. I felt sick and I spat it into the bin. With all the warning signs that I couldn't enjoy bacon anymore, the end of my relationship with bacon was the video of the girl singing to her piglet. Once I'd seen it, suddenly it all made sense and I never tried to eat bacon again. I was also fully aware that had I tried, I wouldn't enjoy the experience whatsoever!

"I could never go vegan because I like bacon too much"

Have you ever heard of a subjective statement before? A subjective statement is based upon personal opinions, assumptions, interpretations, and beliefs. Therefore, it's not always accurate! Newspaper editorials, blogs, biographies, and comments on the internet are all examples of places you're likely to find subjective statements.

On the other hand, objective statements are based on an observation of measurable facts. They can be found in encyclopaedias, textbooks, and news reporting (those that have integrity). So, what we have is two types of statements that are based on different things and referenced differently.

The writings, teaching, findings, references, and content in this book are a combination of subjective and objective information. The subjective and objective statements come from myself and others, from personal experience and online comments.

Usually, a subjective statement is based on events that some people will relate to, and others won't. We are all different after all! However, now you know what a subjective statement is, you'll be able to keep your wits about you when you hear or see one—and make your own mind up!

When you decide to try a vegan diet, one of the things you might hear is "I could never go vegan because I like bacon too much". In fact, many of the things you hear and the misconceptions about vegans is literally just a matter of opinion—based on someone's version of events. From experience, when it comes to your diet, you are much more likely to have to deal with subjective statements from the people around you, rather than objective statements.

Although the liking bacon example isn't the biggest thing in the world to worry about, it is a reason why people may decide not to even try a plant-based diet—or give it a go for more than one attempt. Maybe you even tried a vegan diet before and missed bacon. However, just think of all the things that you and others persisted with before they actually came good. Things get easier over time, and often end up better than what they were before.

Bacon isn't the be all and end all of planet earth (some would disagree mind you!). If you really love bacon, replace it with something else you like and persist with it. This is a beaming example of how far you can go to make your diet more suitable for you in the long run.

What's happening to me?

After the bacon situation, I was keen to continue and press on with life as "normal". This meant eating lots of meat to fulfil my requirements for the "best" sources of protein, which I'm sure we all know, is essential to a healthy lifestyle.

While the bacon thing was going on, not once had I experienced the sick feeling I had eating pig towards any other animal.

My lifestyle at the time was very physically demanding. As well as being relatively flat out physically when it came to coaching clients (1-1 & group fitness), I was also training as often as my time allowed. Without getting too technical, this meant that I had a truly above average demand for protein. My nutrition at the time was very heavily focused around animal products. Not only to quench my thirst for protein, but because in truth, I enjoyed eating it.

There were other reasons why I included meat as a staple in my diet:

- I liked the taste.
- It gave me peace of mind that I was getting enough protein.
- It was relative to my body composition goals at the time (low body fat/high muscle tone).
- It was a comfortable habit.
- I didn't know any better in comparison to plant-based proteins.

At this stage, my staples included chicken breast, chicken thigh, steak, beef mince, turkey, turkey mince, lamb, tuna, salmon, cod, prawns, eggs, cheese, whey protein, milk, and pretty much anything that came from an animal...bar a pig!

The other components of my diet were what the mainstream media refers to as "clean" foods. This included vegetables such as spinach, kale, rocket, tomatoes, potatoes, and sweet potatoes, and some grains such as brown rice, rice, and oats. I rarely ate bread and avoided sweets and sugar (including fruit most of the time), unless I had been exercising in order to "earn it".

Like most responsible wannabe-healthy people, I prepped my food in advance to control what I consumed in times of hunger. I was eating a copious amount of food on a daily basis in comparison to the average person, or even the average gym-goer, and I definitely felt like I warranted it based on my overall energy expenditure through coaching and training.

Aside from the bacon incident, everything seemed normal until one day, I was eating a prepped meal of beef mince, Spanish onion, garlic, rice and tomato, cooked in olive oil. Then, suddenly, about halfway through eating it, I just couldn't chew the mince anymore, though I could eat the rice and vegetables. I thought: "Don't start this again!" But the thought of chewing it was actually making me feel sick. I had to throw it in the bin just to get it out of my sight. It was like the bacon thing all over again. Except this time I had no signs why it was happening.

I continued to try again on other occasions because I desperately wanted the protein, but to no avail. I started panicking. Meat = protein. Protein = good for me. Very important! It was like I was being held ransom to it. I couldn't even bring myself to chew it anymore. What's more, it was a sign of things to come, as the same thing then started happening with other types of red meat, such as steak and lamb.

"I heard that if you cut down your meat intake, you'll need a supplement to replace it"

If you ever start thinking this way, ask yourself: what would the supplement be replacing exactly? Is it micronutrients such as vitamin B12, vitamin B6, zinc, or iron? Is it protein? Or is it all of these? These nutrients are a common mainstream justification for why humans need to eat meat, as if meat is the only place we can get these nutrients from. We also get them from plants.

First, to resolve this misconception, you need to be as specific as possible about what exactly you need to replace. How deficient are you in these nutrients, and how much of them do you need to meet your daily requirements? Then, do some research into the plant-based alternatives where you can get these nutrients, and consume them solely through food if you don't want to take supplements.

However, if you don't get on with the plant-based alternatives—maybe you don't like the taste, or it's impractical—then you may want to supplement your diet with a high dose multivitamin and mineral, or one that covers you for the specific nutrients you need. This should give you peace of mind while you adjust to getting all of your nutrients from plant-based alternatives.

It's also important to clarify the confusion around the word "supplement". The definition of "supplement" is: a thing added to something else in order to complete or enhance it. Many supplements on the market actually say something like "meant to supplement a highly varied diet of whole, unprocessed foods" on the packet. NOT "to replace a highly varied diet of whole, unprocessed foods". In other words, as well as, not instead of. Just imagine putting a plate of plant-based food next to a plate of tablets and powders... Do you think the supplement will do the same thing for you as all that real food?

Of course not. No one is saying you should only consume supplements, but that they should enhance your diet if you need more of these nutrients. In fact, certain types of people are believed to be deficient in some nutrients compared to the average person and so are advised to take a vitamin and/or mineral supplement to account for this, such as:

- Pregnant and breastfeeding women should take vitamin D supplements.
- Women trying to conceive and women in the first 12 weeks of their pregnancy are recommended to take folic acid supplements, which reduce the baby's risk of neural tube defects.
- People aged 65 and over should take vitamin D supplements.
- Children aged 6 months to 5 years should be given a supplement containing vitamins A, C, and D.

If you don't fall into one of these groups of people advised to take them and you're sceptical about supplements, then you might lean towards "superfoods" as an alternative to supplement, but that have similar properties.

Superfoods are defined as: "nutrient-rich food considered to be especially beneficial for health and well-being". A particular type of food becomes marketed as a "superfood" when it's shown to be proportionately higher in vitamins and minerals compared to most other foods. These superfoods can ward off diseases and help you live longer. That said, many foods have their own significant "goodness" in some form or other.

Mainstream superfood examples include: Acai berries, avocado, blueberries, chia seeds, coconut oil, flaxseeds, garlic, goji berries, hemp seeds, kale, maca powder, raw cacao, spirulina, turmeric, walnuts, mushrooms... and many more.

As you'll discover over the course of this book, there are many ways to fulfil your macronutrient and micronutrient requirements through plant-based foods, not just through supplements.

Personally, I had always been inclined to supplement with vitamins, minerals, herbs, and sports supplements even before I adopted a plant-based diet. Going by popular mainstream belief, I should have been feeling deficient and weak when I stopped consuming animal products—yet I didn't.

Casually swapping red meat for nuts, seeds, and nut butters

Naturally, once I had stopped eating red meat, I decided to focus more on the other types of meat, fish, and protein sources. My first port of call was nuts and nut butters. At this stage, they seemed like the way to go, being relatively high in protein and "healthy fats", and majorly accessible and practical compared to red meat.

In the past, I had often bought nuts and nut butters as an accessory to meat in order to boost protein and healthy fats content. So I knew they were high in micronutrients, such as vitamins and minerals, but I hadn't experimented with them or taken much interest before.

Once I took the time to research the finer details of what these foods could do for me, I was shocked, and also in denial about how much better they were for my health and wellbeing compared to red meat. Deep down, I knew it all along, but I was stuck in a routine.

One of the things I did really like about them was the lack of controversy or associated health risks that red meat came with. The only downside was that some people have nut allergies and would have to avoid them. Fortunately, this didn't apply to me.

Seeds came along later for me personally, but looking back now, I don't know why I didn't switch to eating them sooner. Chances are, if you're going to a supermarket or natural health food store to buy nuts, you'll find seeds.

I began to experiment with different combinations at different times of day to keep it interesting. This included an adventurous approach to combining nuts, seeds, and nut butters with different types of vegetables and fruit.

There are some recommendations to consume a 30g portion or a small handful of nuts or nut butters. This equates to approximately:

- 20 almonds.
- 10 Brazil nuts.
- 15 cashews.
- 4 chestnuts.
- 20 hazelnuts.
- 15 macadamias.
- 15 pecans.
- 2 tablespoons of pine nuts.
- 30 pistachio kernels.
- 10 walnuts.
- Small handful of mixed nuts or seeds.

At this stage, I'd eat between five and eight times a day, so once I realised there were nine different types of nuts, five different types of seeds, and at least four different types of nut butters to replace just three different types of red meat that I was eating, I was sold!

Not only could I use the variety to get different types of nutrition, but they were actually more convenient, as there was no cooking required. They wouldn't rot, didn't go out of date quickly, and were far more cost-effective. Wins all round.

"You need red meat in your diet because it's the best source of iron"

Iron helps to metabolise proteins, plays a role in the production of haemoglobin and red blood cells, and helps transport oxygen throughout the body. The benefits of iron consumption include removing various causes of fatigue.

A lack of iron in the diet causes a decrease in red blood cells and haemoglobin in the blood. Iron deficiency anaemia is a worldwide health problem, especially common in young women and children. When anaemia sets in slowly, the symptoms are often vague and may include feeling tired, weak, short of breath, or having poor ability to exercise.

When people deliberate over or decide to eat a plant-based diet, this is a fundamental concern. However, the role of iron is often misunderstood in the mainstream as having a direct effect on blood. This can lead to people assuming that to increase their iron levels, they need to consume blood i.e. meat! Of course, there is iron in meat. But meat isn't the only source of iron.

The current recommended dietary allowance (RDA) for iron is 8.7mg a day for men and 14.8mg a day for women. Lamb breast contains 1.6mg of iron per 100g and beef steak contains 2.9mg. Here are some alternative plant-based sources (per 100g):

- Spinach: 2.7mg.
- Lentils: 3.3mg.
- Soybeans: 5.1mg.

- Chickpeas: 2.9mg.
- Molasses: 3.4mg.

Other sources include most types of beans, tofu, cashew nuts, chia seeds, flaxseed, hemp seeds, pumpkin seeds, kale, dried apricots, dried figs, raisins, quinoa, and fortified breakfast cereal.

The major difference between the animal sources of iron and plant-based ones is whether the iron is 'heme' or 'non-heme':

- Heme iron is derived from haemoglobin, and is found in animal foods that originally contained haemoglobin, such as red meats, fish, and poultry. In these, it makes up around 40% of the iron.
- Non-heme iron makes up around 60% of the iron in animal tissue and all of the iron in plant-based foods such as fruits, veg, grains, nuts, and seeds.

Non-heme iron is notoriously not as well-absorbed by the body as heme iron. Because of this, some might expect that vegans would be prone to developing iron deficiency anaemia, because a plant-based diet contains only non-heme iron. However, studies have found that iron deficiency anaemia is no more common among vegans than meat eaters. It's also thought that heme iron may increase the risk of cancer, stroke, heart disease, and metabolic syndrome.

Clearly, it's more down to the choices of the individual than the diet itself. Despite these findings, vegans and vegetarians should still be aware of foods that are high in iron, techniques to promote iron absorption, and things to avoid to ensure they take their non-heme iron intake to its full potential.

Vitamin C is said to enhance iron absorption, so you should combine plant-based foods that contain iron with those high in vitamin C. As a matter of fact, vegan diets are often higher in vitamin C than the average diet, thanks to the extra fruits and vegetables consumed (based on the individual's diet of course—you have to actually eat the fruit & veg to get the benefits!).

Foods that contain vitamin C include: Papaya, red and yellow peppers, tomatoes, lemons, limes, broccoli, Brussels sprouts, strawberries, guava, pineapple, oranges, grapefruit, kiwi fruit, blackcurrant, redcurrant, chives and kale.

There's also research into things that reduce iron absorption. One study found that tea and coffee may reduce iron absorption by as much as 60% due to tannins. These water-soluble polyphenols are thought to adversely affect iron availability. Some research suggests you'd have to drink more than three strong cups of tea a day to experience this effect, but it's worth noting if you're looking to max your iron absorption.

Feeling wasteful and ungrateful

I was in denial about what was happening to me. So much so that I'd become stubborn. Sometimes, I'd buy beef mince, cook it, and try to eat it—to no avail! Then it got to the stage when cooking these foods didn't feel right. Food was rotting in the fridge until it went out of date, then went into the bin.

This was something I had never done before, and it was all because I couldn't bring myself to cook it, let alone eat it. I could bring myself to buy it though, which was very annoying! So not only was my hard-earned cash going to waste, but so was valuable food that someone else could have eaten.

Around this time, I read a study stating that almost 50% of food thrown away in the UK comes from in the home. Around 7 million tonnes of food and drink are thrown out from each home every year! And more than half of this is food and drink that could have been consumed. Supposedly, the wasted food costs the average UK household £470 each year, an average of around £10 per week. For those with children, it's £700 a year, or £15 a week. With all that in mind, wasting food is...well...a waste!

By this time, I had replaced the majority of my meals with nuts, seeds, nut butters, chicken, eggs, and fish so I had enough protein. But it wasn't long before history repeated itself and chicken naturally followed suit behind bacon, beef, and lamb. Literally the same process ensued:

1. Couldn't finish all the meat in a meal one day.
2. Couldn't finish most of the meat in a meal one day.
3. Couldn't chew the meat and enjoy the flavour.
4. Couldn't bring myself to eat the meat.
5. Couldn't cook the meat, then would leave the meat in the fridge until it went out of date and had to be thrown away.

Fortunately, by this stage, I was aware of the process and was able to make adjustments, such as not buying so much chicken knowing it would go to waste. Whey protein started to make more of an appearance. A lot more than was ideal to be honest, but I had to adapt. The theory at the time was that it offered a 'lean' source of protein, similar to chicken, so it was the suitable alternative in some occasions. Albeit, processed and cold!

The alternatives weren't my first choice, like meat had been originally. However, I knew my knowledge of plant-based foods hadn't grown enough for me to become entirely confident in the change yet. Even so, the fact that the food I bought was all being put to use made me happier and more positive about my nutrition again. I didn't feel wasteful and ungrateful anymore.

"You need to eat meat to build muscle"

For some people, their knowledge on this subject starts and stops here:

Meat = protein.
Protein = builds muscle.
More protein = more muscles.

Let's look at these points before we move on:

Meat = protein. Yes.

Protein is essential for growth and repair in the body. It helps us maintain good health. Protein is made up of amino acids, often referred to as the basic building blocks of all proteins. Our body needs 21 different amino acids to form usable proteins, and it can produce 12 of these amino acids on its own, but it can't produce the remaining 9. These are called essential amino acids and they have to be consumed through our diet. The 9 essential amino acids are: histidine, isoleucine, leucine, lysine, methionine, phenylalanine, threonine, tryptophan, and valine.

Plant-based foods contain protein. However, there is a misunderstanding in the mainstream that you can't get all 21 amino acids from plant-based foods. Hence, why meat is usually seen as the superior choice for protein as it's well-known to contain a full amino acid profile.

Protein = builds muscle. Yes. To an extent.

Protein helps to build muscle only if there is a need to produce more contractile proteins or repair damaged tissues. This happens either when your muscles have to adapt to the stress of exercise by recruiting more contractile proteins to do more work, or from wounds, blunt trauma, and burns.

After you work out, your body repairs or replaces damaged muscle fibres through a cellular process, where it fuses muscle fibres together to form new muscle protein strands or myofibrils. These repaired myofibrils increase in thickness and number to create muscle hypertrophy (growth). Muscle growth occurs whenever the rate of muscle protein synthesis is greater than the rate of muscle protein breakdown. This adaption does not happen while you actually lift the weights though. It occurs while you rest.

More protein = more muscles. Yes. To an extent.

Eating more protein alone doesn't make your muscles grow bigger or faster. The amount you need also changes over your lifetime.

To ensure you're doing your best to grow muscle, muscle protein synthesis must exceed muscle protein breakdown. This means you need to take in adequate sources of protein and carbohydrates to help facilitate the cellular process of rebuilding broken down muscle tissue. However, more isn't always better, as the body converts excess protein into fat for storage or glucose for energy—depending on a variety of complex factors.

In short, sufficient exercise, nutrition, and recovery is what builds muscle—not just meat. There are many well-known sources of plant-based protein from nuts to seeds, beans, pulses, legumes, and vegetables, including (protein value listed per 100g, rounded up or down and as dry weight):

- Almonds: 21g
- Black beans: 21g.
- Broccoli: 3g.
- Cashews: 18g.
- Chia seeds: 17g.
- Chick peas: 9g.
- Edamame beans: 12g.
- Flaxseeds: 18g.
- Green peas: 5g.
- Hemp seeds: 25g.
- Kale: 4g.
- Lentils: 9g.
- Nutritional yeast: 47g.
- Oats: 13g.
- Peanut butter: 22g.
- Pumpkin seeds: 30g.
- Quinoa: 14g.
- Spinach: 3g.

- Spirulina: 57g.
- Sunflower seeds: 21g.
- Tahini: 17g.
- Tempeh: 20g.
- Tofu: 12g.
- Walnuts: 15g.

In order to increase your chances of consuming all 21 amino acids throughout your day, particularly the essential amino acids; it has been said to combine proteins such as these examples with each other (within reason) as well as other plant-based foods—including fruits and vegetables.

Taking research to a new level

At the end of 2015, I made plans to create a nutritional e-book to help people conduct their own natural liver detox. Having become disheartened with the lack of ethical marketing and integrity in the mainstream media around these types of products, I hoped to put together a book of objective information—something that would actually have true value for someone's health and wellbeing. I had no intention of becoming rich out of it, or proclaiming it to be something it wasn't.

It's no secret that in the mainstream, these types of products are often depicted as a "weight loss miracle" or "quick fix". So much so that most of the products out there promising a liver detox are likely to only appeal to people who buy into quick fixes for weight loss. As such, the general vibe is that the majority of these products are a massive "con" and may actually be bad for your health. Sadly, what tends to happen with people who use these products is that they put on more weight than they started with!

Four weeks of solid research went by that were very insightful. I looked at comprehensive university studies, mainstream reports, and blogs to get both sides. Like most things related to health, there was similar and conflicting information among them. The eye-opener from this research was that some of them said that if you wanted to conduct an effective liver detox, you'd have to exclude many things from your diet—including meat. My gut feeling led me to investigate this further, and all of the signs pointed to one main reason: toxins.

Toxins overall a very complex subject, but in short, they are thought to be found externally (outside your body) and created and built up internally (inside you). The main culprits are food, water, the environment, personal care and beauty products, and stress. As well as meat and animal products, toxins also find their way into fruit and vegetables, mainly through pesticides. Fortunately, washing them before eating reduces this.

Canned foods, ready meals, bottled drinks, and other processed foods such as bread and cereals also contain toxins, but these can be reduced by purchasing the least-processed varieties of these foods. Research showed there was more to this detox shebang than just popping a pill or drinking a shake!

"There is no such thing as a detox"

The definition of "detox" is: A process or period of time in which one abstains from or rids the body of toxic or unhealthy substances; detoxification.

The word "abstain" caught my attention—it means: Restrain oneself from doing or enjoying something.

How many detoxes have you come across that focus on what goes in someone's belly, rather than what goes out of their lifestyle, as a detox should? For example, the mainstream weight loss promises, like pop a pill or drink a shake. These aren't about ridding the body of anything, but consuming more.

It's thought that the body can't get back to health until it's had an opportunity to rid itself of toxins. If we want to rid ourselves of toxins, we need to know what the other causes of toxin build-up are. I doubt you'll be surprised by most of them, as it's common sense that most of these are bad for us:

- Alcohol, smoking, and caffeine.
- Lack of sleep and stress.
- Processed food, added sugar, and artificial sweeteners.
- Wheat and gluten (for some people).
- Meat and animal products (including dairy).

All the classics—and then bam! Until my research, I'd never put meat in this category. You may feel the same. And to be fair, when I did consume the others, like coffee; it was 'in moderation' as my gut told me that too much could have a potentially adverse effect. But not meat. Meat was the "natural" one, or so I thought. The more the merrier. More protein = better, right?

I thought to myself: WTF is it doing on that list with all that other shit! It's a hard pill to swallow when its consumption is seen to be normal in modern society. Associated research pointed to the fact that meat and dairy products are loaded with toxic substances such as antibiotics, growth hormones, pus, accumulated poisons, artery-clogging fat, and more grim stuff.

A few reports stated that sometimes when a person stops consuming meat, their body goes into cleansing (or detox) mode, as it begins to rid itself of accumulated toxins. A number of side effects may occur during this process, such as mild headaches, fatigue, weakness, slight dizziness, mucous drainage, diarrhoea, pimple outbreaks, etc. It's weird to think that abstaining from meat consumption has its own version of going cold turkey. Especially when eating meat is meant to be the normal, natural thing to do!

Initially, reducing your meat intake is your way of 'abstaining', as you may enjoy eating it at the moment. But, if you're like me, you may much prefer the feeling of not having those toxins in your system, and over time, you may want to go fully plant-based.

So, if anyone ever tells you "there is no such thing as a detox", then ask them to define detox. Chances are they're so far on the hate bandwagon that they've never even looked into what it really means. They're probably referring to products that go in your body, as opposed to those you abstain from.

Meat is everywhere!

At a seminar I attended on positive mindset, the speaker told everyone to close their eyes and not think about a pink elephant in the corner of the room. Then he asked everyone to open their eyes and put their hand up if they'd thought about the pink elephant. 100% of people put their hand up.

I wasn't avoiding meat or trying not to think about it, but I was definitely noticing it more than ever before. Although it had obviously been this way for a long time before I'd stopped eating it, I was shocked to see that meat was literally everywhere in society.

At times, I'd go to the supermarket and see that the majority of their advertising was huge banners of meat in traditional meals such as roast dinners, English breakfasts, and burgers—often with blood oozing out, which I found rather unnecessary and gross now! Or I'd go to a restaurant with friends and the majority of the menu was dishes with meat. Or I'd go to grab a sandwich on the go and literally all of them contained meat or animal products. The list was endless. It was like a gauntlet—I couldn't escape the fucking stuff!

Every nutritional decision I made in these moments went against the grain of what was the most accessible and "traditional" in modern society. If I didn't think it would be worth the effort, then I would have cracked on and eaten meat at this point. But from the beginning, I always said to myself that if something felt natural, then I would keep doing it. If it didn't, then I wouldn't. In this case, not eating meat felt natural, so I was going to keep doing that.

I was actually in disbelief that meat had become the more convenient and accessible option—given the fact that killing an animal, skinning it, and gutting it seemed like a lot more hassle than just picking something off a tree or out of the ground! Questions revolved in my head about why this was the case. It also made me feel a bit "weird", like I was different to everyone else for not eating it, and for thinking that a huge banner of a burger oozing blood was unnecessary while nobody else seemed to even notice it!

When you look into the history of eating meat, humans have apparently been eating and hunting animals for about 2.5 million years, going by fossil records. As such, I can understand why there is this mentality to glorify dead things, why it's acceptable and even "normal" to most people. So much so that nobody even bats an eyelid to it. So, I accepted the fact that it's just the way it is because that's just the way it's always been.

"White meat is better for you than red meat"

In general, red meats such as beef, pork, and lamb are thought to have more cholesterol and saturated fat than white meats such as chicken and fish, which is why white meat is usually depicted as better for you in the mainstream. However, this isn't exclusively true. Some foods can have a relatively high amount of cholesterol and very little saturated fat at the same time.

Cholesterol plays a vital role in how every cell works and it's also needed to make vitamin D, some hormones, and bile for digestion. It's a waxy substance made inside us by the liver, but it's also found in meat and offal (liver, kidneys, etc), prawns, crab, lobster, squid, octopus, and eggs. All animal products contain cholesterol.

Cholesterol is carried in the blood attached to proteins called lipoproteins. There are two main forms: LDL (low density lipoprotein) and HDL (high density lipoprotein):

- LDL cholesterol is often referred to as "bad cholesterol", because it's the main source of artery-clogging plaque. Too much of this type of cholesterol in the blood can increase your risk of heart and circulatory diseases.
- HDL is often referred to as "good cholesterol", because of its protective benefits. It attempts to clear the "bad" from the blood and prevent heart disease and sudden attacks such as stroke.

Up to 2015, the recommendation for total dietary cholesterol per day was 300mg– or 200 mg if you had a high risk of heart disease. At this present time there are no specific recommended limits for the amount of cholesterol you consume from food. That being said, it's still important to pay attention to the food you eat in order to keep your body's cholesterol levels in a healthy range. This includes limiting your intake of saturated fats, trans-fats and added sugars.

There are no known plant-based foods that contain cholesterol. One large boiled chicken egg (50g) contains almost 200mg of cholesterol. Let's take a look at other popular foods and their cholesterol (all per 100g):

- Bacon, fried: 99mg.
- Pulled pork: 35mg.
- Beef, mince: 88mg.
- Beef, steak: 79mg.
- Chicken breast: 75mg.
- Chicken thigh: 90mg.
- Lamb leg shank: 88mg.
- Lamb breast: 103mg.
- Cod: 55mg.
- Salmon: 71mg.
- Tuna, bluefin: 30mg.
- Mackerel: 59mg.
- Prawn: 189mg.

Having too much saturated fat in your diet can raise "bad" cholesterol in the blood, which increases the risk of heart disease and sudden attacks. It's worth nothing that there are different types of fat ("good" and "bad"), such as monounsaturated and polyunsaturated. We'll focus on the "bad" stuff for now—in particular saturated fat and trans-fat. We'll get into the "good" stuff later in the book.

The current RDA for saturated fat is no more than 30g a day for men and no more than 20g for women. It's thought that the UK population gets around 13% of their daily energy (calories) from saturated fats on average, which is slightly above the 11% recommended maximum. Here are the same foods from our previous list, but with their saturated fat level (all per 100g):

- Bacon, fried: 12g.
- Pulled pork: 1g.
- Beef, mince: 6g.
- Beef, steak: 6g.
- Chicken breast: 2g.
- Chicken thigh: 4g.
- Lamb leg shank: 5g.
- Lamb breast: 16.8g.
- Cod: 0g.
- Salmon: 1g.
- Tuna, bluefin: 1g.
- Mackerel: 10g.
- Prawn: 0g.

Bad saturated fat is the mostly solid type of fat, and it's found in foods such as butter, lard, pies, cakes, biscuits, fatty cuts of meat, sausages, bacon, cheese, cream, and palm and coconut oil. You could say that bad saturated fat is evidently found in junk food containing animal products. This is excluding palm and coconut oil, which are plant-based, but these also appear in junk foods alongside animal products or as an alternative for something else.

If you eat any of these junk foods, you could also be consuming another type of bad saturated fat– trans-fats. These are also found in deep fried foods, biscuits, cakes, and pastries. They're mainly produced by an industrial process called hydrogenation, and can be spotted as "hydrogenated oils". Trans-fats are evidently found in junk food containing animal products. There are no known plant-based foods that contain trans-fats.

Trans-fats, like most saturated fats, raise blood cholesterol levels, particularly levels of "bad" cholesterol. They can also reduce the "good" cholesterol, and increase another form of blood fat called triglycerides. All of the effects of trans-fats can raise your risk of coronary heart disease (CHD). Gram for gram, trans-fats appear to increase our risk of CHD more than saturated fats, and therefore are potentially worse for our health. As such, you should avoid trans-fats where possible.

The UK doesn't participate in as much trans-fat activity as the U.S., but keep an eye out for–and avoid–hydrogenated oils in food where possible. Recommendations are that trans-fat consumption shouldn't exceed 2% of food energy overall. For a 2000-calorie overall daily intake, this equates to only 40 calories–literally a minuscule amount. For most people, a quick fix to reduce their saturated fat and trans-fat consumption is to eat less animal products and junk foods, or avoid eating them entirely.

Casually swapping cow's milk for plant-based milk

I've never been the type of person who drinks a glass of milk straight. Mind you, as an Englishman, I love a cup of tea! Though it usually only consisted of a drop of milk anyway. I never used milk on my porridge, just boiling water, and sweetened it with fruit. So, naturally, it wasn't that hard to make the switch. I began drinking more herbal tea and black coffee instead of white.

Some might say that I was jumping the gun en route to a plant-based diet, as cow's milk is widely acceptable for vegetarians. However, it felt completely like the natural thing for me to do at this stage. The catalyst for the change was stumbling across an article on the effects of dairy on the body. It gave an insight into the hormones and toxins found in cow's milk, and I concluded that these things probably aren't best-suited for human consumption.

Seeing a video of pus on a cow's udder also helped to speed up my switch from cow's milk. What's more, during my research, some of the content referred to cow's milk as "pregnant cows' breast milk", and "liquid flesh". I might as well be honest about my feelings—it fucking freaked me out! Interestingly, you think I would have made the connection to other dairy products at this point, but somehow I was still able to eat cheese, chocolate, and whey protein without thinking twice, even though milk grossed me out.

I quickly found out there are many different types of plant-based milk including almond, cashew, coconut, hazelnut, hemp, oat, rice, pea, and soy. Also, I was shocked by how much nicer they were than cow's milk! I kept it really basic early on, being more familiar with almond milk than the alternatives. But as time went by, I regularly changed it up and actually looked forward to trying a new flavour or brand—as they were all delicious.

Naturally, I came across other varieties of these milks, including organic, sweetened or unsweetened versions, chocolate editions, and even hybrids such as coconut mixed with almond. This made it even easier to choose the alternatives over cow's milk.

I also came to the realisation that plant-based milk isn't just bought by vegans, but by those who are lactose-intolerant (among other conditions) or who just prefer it, be it for taste or peace of mind. Unlike its animal-based counterpart, plant-based milk contains no lactose or cholesterol, so it's more fitting for those with certain health conditions.

Nutritionally, plant-based milk tends to vary, mostly dependant on the supplier. One thing is rather consistent though—they are often fortified with micronutrients, such as added calcium and vitamin B12. "Fortified" basically means they have had these things added to them, similar to what you see in cereals and supplements. By contrast, cow's milk doesn't usually contain these added nutrients.

When I weighed all of this up, for the first time in my life I actually looked forward to drinking a glass of milk. I even started using it in my porridge from time to time. Even better, other than soya milk, I didn't suffer from any digestive problems or get that weird milk coating in the back of my throat from drinking dairy products. It was another win-win to add to my growing collection of plant-based alternatives.

"You need cow's milk in your diet because it's the best source of calcium"

In 2005, Britain had more than 14,500 dairy farms. One year later, there were just over 9,500 left. Like any industry, milk is a business and it works on supply and demand. The more you want, the more they produce. And vice versa. Back in the day, people clearly wanted more milk than they do now, and farmers have faced an increasing drop in demand as time goes by.

From my research into milk, I have to say that those responsible for marketing the dairy industry back in the day were amazing—way ahead of their time! They were the pioneers of "healthy" nutrition in the mainstream, and you've got to give them credit, given the fact that what they were marketing comes from a pregnant cow. Not something you'd think would be that attractive. They made it "normal" and even desirable in society.

Unfortunately, the information that's so accessible online now wasn't available back then. These days, people are clocking onto more superior plant-based sources of calcium. As a result, they're are going for alternatives instead.

The current RDA for adults aged 18-64 is 700mg per day. Whole fat cow's milk contains 113mg per 100g. Here are some sources of calcium from plant-based foods per 100g:

- Unhulled sesame seeds: 975mg.
- Tahini: 426mg.
- Tofu: 267mg.
- Almonds: 269mg.
- Collard greens: 232mg.

Other sources of calcium include: molasses, dandelion greens, black eyed peas, seaweed, rocket, kale, watercress, spinach, hazelnuts, pak choi, okra, sunflower seeds, broccoli, and oranges.

The last time I ate meat ... Ever!

My desire to eat any meat whatsoever was non-existent at this stage, though I was eating more fish. I had also completely phased out cow's milk. So, when I broke the seal and ate meat again, it really did come as a surprise.

One of my all-time favourite meals (pre-plant-based days) was my mum's chicken fajitas. Having got back late from work one night, exhausted and hungry, I walked into the kitchen to make some dinner. I was thinking of cooking some rigatoni, rocket, tomato, avocado, and tuna with sunflower seeds. Sorted. But my idea was side-tracked when I noticed a foil-covered bowl on the worktop with a note beside it:

Glen,
Have left you bowl of leftovers from chicken fajitas earlier.
Wasn't sure if you wanted any or not.
Other stuff you will need is in fridge.
You can have all of it.

The message was left by my sister, and I really appreciated it. This kind of thing rarely happened and when it did, I would usually be over the moon. Let's face it—who can turn down free food? Let alone your favourite meal of all time, already cooked up and conveniently left on the side for you with an inviting note! Plus, the thought of having to cook from scratch wasn't welcoming. It was late, and I was exhausted.

However, it was too good to be true. Firstly, my mouth wasn't exactly salivating at the thought of eating meat again. I debated sticking to my guns and not eating it. It felt like a test on my quest to a plant-based diet. I thought: "Do you really want to never eat chicken fajitas again?" But I had a strong gut feeling that it would be a short-lived high, mostly on the taste buds for old time's sake, and would leave me feeling a bit sick after it. On the flip side, I knew from the previous times that throwing food away left me feeling wasteful and ungrateful. Basically, I was fucked either way!

I decided to listen to my childhood nostalgia feeling over my gut feeling. I built the chicken fajitas up the way I always had done. I ate them, regretting each bite as I went, but determined to not let any to go to waste. Once I had eaten them, I felt instant regret, as if what I had done was morally wrong for a number of reasons:

- I was in the process of structuring a book on how people could go about adhering to a plant-based diet. Fail.
- I was lying to myself that I had actually taken in any of the research I had recently gathered. Fail.
- I already knew that eating meat felt completely pointless and weird to me at this stage. Fail.

The taste, texture, and eating experience was nowhere near what I remembered. It was completely different now—and eating meat didn't feel natural to me at all. In all honesty, I was pretty certain that I would never eat meat ever again before this happened. But you know what they say: "Old habits die hard."

I didn't cry about this situation though. I tried to learn from it. From this point on, I never made the same mistake again. I kept my nutritional choices in sync with my gut feeling at the time—always going with what felt like the most natural thing to do.

"Humans have canines, which means that they must be designed to eat meat"

The differentiability between the renowned characteristics of any type of animal can be classified through the foods that they primarily eat. Be it meat, plant-based foods, or a combination of both.

Natural physiology is a deciding factor in what foods an animal should be consuming in the long term i.e. what their digestive system can handle and what effects these foods will have on their health. However, another form of identification involves natural instinct in the animal's preferred choice of food. This means whether they have a natural disposition for a particular food group—not just in order to survive, but to thrive.

For humans, this is a little different to most animals, since we can source any type of food we want (for the majority in the Western world anyway), simply by clicking a button to order it to our door. Or waltz into a supermarket. Animals, on the other hand, often have to take what they can get to reach tomorrow—they can't be so fussy.

There are three main ways that an animal is distinguished physiologically, based on their dietary requirements to thrive:

- Carnivore: An animal that feeds on other animals.
- Omnivore: An animal that eats a variety of food from both plant and animal origin.
- Herbivore: An animal that feeds on plants.

Now, people often assume that because humans have canines, we must therefore share similar traits and dietary requirements with other animals that also have canines. A canine tooth can be easily identified, as it is the longer, pointed tooth located on either side of the incisors, and it is often greatly enlarged in carnivores.

In the uninformed imagination, most people think of animals with canines are being carnivorous species such as big cats, which only feed on other animals. And bears, which feed on both animals and plants, and so are classified as omnivores. Most people are also well-aware that humans eat a variety of plant and animal food. So, we must therefore be omnivores. And omnivores also have canines, like carnivores. Therefore, we must be designed to eat meat. Right?

Unfortunately, the answer to this question isn't that simple. Canines are just the tip of the iceberg in this popular reasoning. Firstly, having canines alone doesn't rubber-stamp which category a species falls into. If this was the case, gorillas would be blatantly omnivorous, because they have massive canines. Yet, they exclusively feed and thrive off plant foods for their whole lifetimes.

So, if gorillas aren't designed to eat meat purely because they have canines, why would humans be?! What's more, in comparison to a gorilla's canines, a human's canines are pretty minuscule!

Canines in general across the three main types (plus humans):

- Carnivore: Great sharp fangs.
- Omnivore: Great sharp fangs.
- Herbivore: Undeveloped in comparison, short and blunted.
- Human: Undeveloped in comparison, short and blunted.

It's worth noting that while the presence of canines does not guarantee an animal is a carnivore, it is an indicator that meat may be some part of its diet. This is because carnivores use their teeth to kill their prey before eating it. However, the presence of canines alone as an indicator of something being a carnivore is simply a common misconception.

Eating meat ... It's a culture thing

If you pay any attention to social media, you'll remember a story a while back about a lion being shot in Africa. 'Cecil the Lion' grabbed the attention of the internet, with people in complete dismay and disgust at the news. I recall people saying they wanted to do some pretty bad things to the man who killed Cecil. Everyone was talking about it, and it seemed like everyone had the same views on the situation. That being: it was morally wrong to kill a lion.

Around the same time, there was another discussion regarding animal welfare, in which everyone seemed to share the same views of disgust—the annual dog meat festival in China. There were petitions going around online, and I remember how many people were outraged by this. It was abundantly clear how many people thought it was morally wrong to eat a dog.

One day, I was lying on my bed pondering this subject when my cat Bruce jumped up beside me and started doing that cat thing of getting in your personal space. I have always shamelessly admitted that Bruce is one of my best friends. I petted him for a while, then he went and sat at the end of my bed near my feet, looking back at me. As I was looking at him, the thought crossed my mind: "I wonder whether people eat cats too...?" With that in mind, I did some research and found that, yes, humans do in fact eat cats in some Asian countries!

As you can imagine, the thought of this horrified me. Bruce is one of my best friends of all time and I love him dearly. He's such a nice bloke, how could anyone ever eat someone like him? Then I thought more logically about the festival going on and realised festival = celebration. People are actually celebrating this! To the people celebrating in China, this is "normal". My research also led me to understand that not everyone in China feels this way, as some people have dogs as pets and don't support the festival.

For the first time, I saw the inconsistency in preference surrounding the meat that people eat, how some people agree with eating certain types, and how some do not—all from a moral standpoint. I also saw those in my own culture react to someone else's dietary preferences in a negative way, as if it were disgusting and inhumane. There was an obvious difference between cultures, which before had not seemed so obvious.

I thought about the conventional Western diet overall. For a culture that eats a lot of different types of meat, it seemed strange as there are no qualms over eating farm animals such as pigs, cows, lambs, and chickens—in their droves. Talk about being hypocritical!

Then I thought about religion, as this also affects how a culture behaves. For example, followers of Judaism and Islam don't eat pork, and followers of Hinduism often don't eat beef. When I started piecing all of this logic together, I realised that the meat you eat is based on your culture—and not on what is morally right or wrong, because what is right to your culture could be wrong to the next. Both culturally and morally.

To get further insight, I looked into some local statistics on attitude towards cats and dogs. The UK pet population in 2015 was estimated at around 20 million (excluding fish) and it's thought that 50% of households own a pet. An estimated 8.5 million of these are dogs, and 7.4 million cats. Even though those in the UK wouldn't eat these types of animals, the RSPCA investigate more than 140,000 complaints of cruelty and neglect every year to animals. Sadly, around 5,000 stray dogs are put to sleep a year, equating to around 14 a day. Some reports suggest that this number is actually far greater.

Overall, there seemed to be major inequality in how animals are treated compared to other animals simply based on human traditions and culture. Even in the UK. It just didn't make sense to me that animals were being treated badly, regardless of whether they were going to become meat or not. It all seemed so unjust.

One thing was for sure, I was certain that I no longer wanted to be part of this animal inequality and favouritism. It lacked consistency, with no real evidence that we should or shouldn't eat one type of animal for any particular reason. Other than religious beliefs, which could be subjective for the individual. I decided that the only way forward was to treat all animals with the same respect and not put the types above one another.

The scary thing was that I thought to myself, had I have been born in China, I may have eaten dog at some point. Or had I born in certain parts of Asia, I would have probably tried cat meat before!

"I've grown up eating meat and animal products, so I don't understand why I should stop now"

You'll be surprised just how commonly this occurs. But what you'll come to realise is this is a premeditated excuse why giving up meat and animal products is pretty much impossible–without even trying.

When some people feel the urge to not eat animals, without even trying to find out more, they instead head-fuck themselves and eat meat every day. All the while fantasising about what it would be like to not eat it! Just because they've always eaten meat, so why change?

Your gut feeling to change is a representation of your body, mind, and senses having a conversation about you. It is in your jurisdiction to eavesdrop on this conversation and act accordingly. Even if it's only for a trial period. And regardless of your past habits and preferences.

Just because you've always done something doesn't mean you need to keep doing it if something is telling you that a change is due.

For example:

- In 2015, the World Health Organisation (WHO) warned that processed meat such as sausages, bacon, and ham can cause cancer, and that red meat likely causes cancer. As a result, 29% of people in the UK apparently reduced their meat consumption. A further 9% were reported to be considering reducing their meat intake or cutting it out entirely. (British Social Attitude survey 2016).

- Some 58% of UK residents cutting back on meat said they were doing so for health reasons, while around 20% were trying to save money, and another 20% were concerned about animal welfare or food safety.

While these statistics don't consider whether people were considering switching to a vegetarian or vegan diet, people may be heading that way whether they realise or not, going by mainstream and social recognition of nutritional preferences.

Bottom line, it's never too late to create change. Even if change can be scary; the unknown!

I wish I ate less meat

Like the pink elephant situation before when I started to notice meat everywhere, there was a time when I kept hearing people talk about their desire to eat less meat. It was really interesting to hear insights that people wanted to reduce their meat consumption.

For the first time, I was starting to learn more about everything— just from speaking to people first-hand about their views. In comparison to the medical journals, documentaries, and seminars, I can honestly say that speaking to people was equally as important in helping me understand the process. I spoke to different types of people—men, women, all ages, all backgrounds.

When I spoke to people about why they wanted to reduce their meat intake, some said it was for their health, because they'd heard that meat was bad for them. Some wanted to do it for the environment, because they'd heard about the knock-on effects of animal agriculture on global warming and thought it was unfair for younger generations. Some people wanted to eat less meat because of how cruel it was for the animals, and because they didn't agree with the meat and dairy industries full stop.

Despite the different reasons for people wanting to reduce their meat consumption, there were a few consistencies that came up too. Some of these opinions may resonate with your own. People felt:

- They needed some meat in their diet, even a bit, to get enough protein.
- They shouldn't eat red meat often, because it can cause cancer.
- That white meat is better for us.
- They wanted to reduce their meat consumption (or stop altogether), but didn't want to become "one of those vegans" because that would be "taking it too far".
- There's no point in eating meat alternatives such as veggie sausages, because "what's the point?"
- Most commonly, they didn't know how to do it and were scared that it could go wrong.

At the time, I hadn't spoken to anyone about phasing out my meat consumption with the intention of switching to a fully plant-based diet one day. Or that I was putting together research to write a book. I wanted to keep learning from as many different sources as possible without coming across as biased when having an open conversation.

I was actually shocked by some people's admissions on why they wanted to make the change. It was clear that many people had given it a thought, but were just lacking the confidence and direction to execute it.

"There's no point reducing my meat intake because one person isn't going to make much of a difference"

This is a really common thing I hear when someone is explaining why they aren't considering the idea further. Let's just look at some figures:

- Over 56 billion farm animals are killed every year by humans worldwide.
- These figures don't include fish and other sea creatures, whose deaths are so huge in number that they are only measured in tonnes.
- Over a billion animals were killed in UK slaughterhouses alone in 2013.
- This included 9.8 million pigs. Nearly 15 million sheep. 18 million turkeys. 14 million ducks. Over 945 million chickens. 2.6 million cattle.
- Add to that 4.5 billion fish and 2.6 billion shellfish— and that's a total of over 8 billion animals killed in the UK each year.
- This equates to around 22 million animals slaughtered every day.

Now, the average UK resident is reported to consume on average two-thirds less meat than the average U.S. resident. But, even the U.S. has seen a decline in meat consumption and an increase in people proactively reducing their meat intake.

Meat consumption has been steadily declining in the U.S. by 10% per person since 2007. The knock-on effect of this that in 2007, the U.S. raised and killed 9.5 billion land animals for food, but in 2014, that decreased by 400 million. You can scale that number down for the UK to get the idea. In essence, you eat less meat personally, and less animals are killed. Less demand, less production.

While the number of reported vegetarians in the U.S. has stayed the same (at around 5%-8% of the population) for years, the number of people reducing their meat intake is fuelling this reduction in animals being killed. This demonstrates that just because someone might not class themselves as a vegetarian or vegan, it doesn't mean they're not making a difference.

These figures show a collective statistic brought about over time and volume. However, to break it down to you personally and the impact you can have, it's important to remember that every individual makes a difference, and each stage towards your plant-based diet will have a greater impact.

One thing is for sure. Whatever you do, no matter how seemingly small or how slowly you move towards your plant-based diet, will ever be a wasted effort. Your decision to not consume animal products will have a big knock-on effect around the world to places and things besides just you. We'll get into the other benefits later in the book.

It's time for change

I decided I was going to own up and speak openly about my nutritional preferences to other people in conversation. It turns out that I'd had a "nutritional title" since the start of the process. Someone who reduces their meat consumption is commonly known as a "flexitarian" or "reduceatarian".

The definition of a flexitarian is something like this: A person who has a primarily vegetarian diet but occasionally eats meat or fish.

The definition of a reduceatarian is something like this: A person who mindfully reduces their meat and fish intake to merge with their beliefs.

The definition of pescatarian is something like this: A person who does not eat meat but does eat fish.

I already knew what a "pescatarian" was from my involvement in the fitness industry, though I hadn't met or had to cater for many during my career. On my plant-based journey, my natural instinct had led me to this title. Although I don't think a nutritional title is completely necessary, it can help you understand your preferences and boundaries in society.

Once I had owned up to the title of pescatarian, the smallest things in day-to-day life became easier. For example, I knew where to focus my attention when it came to food shopping and eating out... on fish! If I ever had a conversation about meat with someone, I already knew how I would explain my nutritional preferences. Funnily enough, many people I spoke to already knew what a pescatarian diet entailed and completely accepted it.

"If you're low on energy when you've dropped meat and animal products from your diet, it's because you need to eat meat and animal products for energy"

Whenever you drop something from your diet and don't replace or substitute it with something else of more or the equivalent amount of energy (calories), you create a reduction in overall energy intake (calorie intake) for the day. This is true for anything, not just meat.

Let's say you have an average daily calorie intake of 2500kcal, which you've calculated as your 'maintenance' calories plus your energy expenditure through activity. Let's say this amount keeps your weight and energy levels stable, and you feel you can perform everything optimally and consistently. Physically and mentally, you feel "just right". Sounds good, yeah?

Now let's throw a spanner in the works. You consume meat, fish, or animal products with three of your meals: breakfast, lunch, and dinner. You often enjoy "hearty", home-cooked meals as opposed to buying food out. You believe this is better for you, and that you have a good balance.

So, you decide to stop eating meat and animal products altogether, but you don't replace them with anything and just go about your meals as normal. Common sense should tell you this isn't the right way to go about it, as you need to eat more of the other stuff or find a suitable replacement. But let's assume you don't know this, so we can understand this common misconception.

- In the morning, you eat a fry-up of bacon, egg, mushrooms, and baked beans with coconut oil: 2 slices of bacon = 112kcal. 2 fried eggs = 202kcal. Total reduction = 313kcal.

- At lunchtime, you eat pre-prepped baked chicken breast, chorizo, and penne pasta salad with honey mustard dressing: 160g chicken breast = 277kcal. 20g chorizo = 91kcal. Total reduction = 368kcal.

- At dinner, you eat a home-cooked meal of chilli con carne, including lean beef mince (5% fat), with kidney beans, rice, aubergine, sweetcorn, and tomato sauce, with a handful of cheddar cheese on top: 100g beef mince = 174kcal. 30g cheddar cheese = 121kcal. Total reduction = 295kcal.

Then we add up the total calories from these three meals, which equates to 976kcal (rounded up to 1000kcal for explanation purposes). Let's say you remove all of these from your average daily diet at once. This provides your new daily average calorie intake of 2500kcal - 1000kcal = 1500kcal.

Obviously, if you were functioning optimally before, then suddenly dropping 1000kcal will be highly noticeable in your energy levels. Without replacing those 1000kcal in the form of other foods, that's nearly half of the total amount you were eating. That's 40% of your energy! You're left with a deficit of 1000kcal against your maintenance weight (plus energy expenditure through activity), meaning you've created a caloric deficit, which is essential if someone wants to lose weight.

However, even a 40% reduction in calories over an extended period of time is quite steep in my book. If someone told me they wanted to lose weight and reduce body fat, in most cases I'd recommend a small reduction in calories and extending the process over a longer duration. For example, a 5-10% calorie reduction long term, until they reach their target weight or target body fat percentage.

There's a good reason for this: a sudden, extreme reduction in calorie intake against energy expenditure, whether accidental (like in being naive in our example) or on purpose (such as to lose weight) can promote eating disorders, spin off into other extreme diets, and in some cases lead to malnutrition, health problems, and needing medical treatment. What's more, in the long run, the weight often goes back on faster than it was to lose!

Malnutrition is defined as: A lack of proper nutrition, caused by not having enough to eat, not eating enough of the right things, or being unable to use the food that one does eat. Symptoms of malnutrition include unintentional weight loss, a low body weight (going by BMI), lack of interest in eating or drinking, feeling tired all the time, feeling weaker, getting ill often, and taking a long time to recover.

Fortunately, in this day and age there are top-notch apps and websites that tell us how many calories, macronutrients, and micronutrients we should be eating to reach our goals. MyFitnessPal is the most famous, the most user-friendly, and a great place to start working out your daily caloric balance and macronutrient totals. You can also use it to familiarise yourself with how your current and past food choices affect your daily totals. I highly recommend you start using this app asap (**find it at myfitnesspal.com**).

There's another app named Cronometer, which covers more in-depth compartments of your nutrition such as micronutrients and amino acids, but stick with MyFitnessPal for now and we'll get into Cronometer later on.

The best thing about these apps is that they're becoming more and more specific to the user. All you have to do is follow the steps, enter your details where prompted, and it does all of the calculations for you. It considers your age, gender, weight, height, daily activity levels, and weight goals, then generates a target number of daily calories for you to reach your desired weight. You have to choose whether you want to lose, maintain or gain and this choice will affect the total calories you'll be aiming for.

For the purpose of this example, we'll say you've chosen to maintain your current weight. You input or search for the foods you've eaten that day in the in-app database and the app will subtract the total for each meal from your total daily calorie aim. If you consume more than your target calories, you'll be in surplus, which will lead to weight gain if you keep it up over an extended period. If you consume less than your target calories, you'll be in deficit, which will lead to weight loss if you keep it up over an extended period.

If you want to eat more than your target amount without putting on weight, you can tinker with the guidelines by doing more exercise and then inputting/searching for the activity in the database. It will account for the total calories burned during the activity and will gift you with those calories on top of your total amount. You can also do this if you want to create a greater caloric deficit but don't want to starve yourself.

Say you've dropped meat and some animal products from your diet. You should consider all of these questions if you are feeling low on energy having dropped animal products from your diet:

- Does this equate to a caloric deficit against your total maintenance number of calories?
- If yes, have you replaced these calories with other calories?
- If yes, then what is the quality of these calories?
- Have you replaced the meat and animal products with

more varied and nutritious plant-based foods? Or have you just increased the amount of the foods you're eating now?

- Have you worked out your maintenance number of calories against your energy expenditure through an app such as MyFitnessPal?

Seasonal deficiency is also possible if someone is low on energy after they've dropped meat and animal products. For example, I tend to eat more stodgy foods such as bread in the winter vs. nutritional foods such as salads. So, remember to look after your vitamin and mineral intake all year round.

A suitable, plant-based replacement for animal products calorie-wise in the short term should keep you on form before you adapt and adjust your macronutrient ratios to your goals.

You could also match the protein and fat levels in plant-based foods with the foods you're replacing. Fat is much higher in calories than protein and carbohydrate—pretty much double the calories per 1g. So, a lot of the calories now missing from your diet may have come from meat and animal products before. These products are often cooked in oil, which is the most fat-dense food, so a meat-eater's calories are being bumped up everywhere!

Let's say you're already on a plant-based diet, living at your maintenance calories, and decide you're not going to eat bread anymore because you heard it's bad for you. But you don't want to lose weight. You normally eat four slices a day, which is around 400kcal. Have you considered what you'll replace this with to account for the 400kcal you're missing out on daily? Maybe you eat four pieces of fruit instead, thinking it's a straight swap, carb for carb. But this might not amount to the same daily total calories, creating a calorie deficit. This might lead to ongoing weight loss and less energy for the foreseeable future.

It's worth noting that you could feel like shit at any time, on any diet, even if you eat your maintenance calories. The reason for this is purely choosing to eat junk food that's low on micronutrients most of the time. A little heads-up: add more nutritious foods such fruits, vegetables, nuts, seeds, beans, legumes, and grains and you'll have more energy.

REDUCE summary

Stop eating a certain type of meat altogether.

The first one you pick could be for a number of reasons, like it's your least favourite taste, or a gut feeling that it may not be right for you. You needn't be too picky, as eventually you may stop eating all types.

Trust your gut feeling.

Once you've acknowledged that something has changed, your body and mind will often have a conversation about what is naturally best for you. It's in your best interests to eavesdrop on this conversation and trust your gut... Literally!

Swap red meat for nuts, seeds, and nut butters.

Doing this will provide a fitting protein and fat source, which may be of similar overall calorie content to what you had before. This will allow you to balance your energy levels more accordingly at the beginning.

Open your mind to new research.

Take everything you already believe to be true about food and then imagine you're learning from scratch. Reserve no judgement about your new findings and keep an open mind while you proactively seek the actual facts. The effect of toxins are a good place to start.

Do not trust the media, both mainstream and social media.

If you want to get the best information and research available, you'll have to go above and beyond society's norm. Look to the top medical professionals and advocates who've covered this subject and make your own judgement from there.

Look into doing something like a "meat-free Monday".

If you're dead set on heading towards a plant-based diet, you could experience what it's like by having one day per week where you go meat-free or fully plant-based. Which day you decide on will depend on your schedule.

Swap meat for meat-based alternatives if you want to.

What's the most obvious replacement for meat in your diet? That would be a meat-based alternative! One that looks, smells, and even tastes like the real thing. That said, like the real thing, they aren't the healthiest thing to eat either. You may like them though.

Swap plant-based milk for cow's milk.

Learn to love it. Embrace the change and get to know as many flavours and brands as possible. If you can subliminally train yourself to drink milk so casually over the years, chances are you could do the same with a more suitable alternative.

Switch up your morning routine.

Starting your day with a plant-based alternative can kickstart new habits from the off and set the tone for the whole day. If it's cereal and/or coffee for example, you could replace milk with water or a plant-based alternative.

Eat meat if you want to.

You'll know how you feel during and after whether it was a good idea or not! Try not to let yourself get "cut short" when it comes to eating for convenience. Set aside some time each week to prep your food in advance to avoid eating things you may regret.

Use MyFitnessPal to track your calorie and macronutrient intake.

The best insights you can get on whether you're meeting your daily nutrient targets is by tracking your food intake with an app.

Stage Two

PESCATARIAN

Trying all things fishy

Some people don't class fish as animals, and from my own experience, at this stage I certainly saw no moral wrong-doing in eating fish, or any seafood for that matter. It's not that I didn't want to stop eating fish, but I genuinely had no urgency or desire to do so right away. At the time, I didn't feel any attachment or connection to fish like I did with land animals. I'd come across research about fish, but I couldn't attach the feeling of unjust inequality to them like I'd done for land animals.

So, perhaps this stage of the process was a bit unconventional compared to most people en-route to a plant-based diet, but instead of immediately trying to phase out fish, I ate more fish and seafood alongside steamed vegetables. The reason was that it felt like the 'natural' thing to do at the time.

I also began to buy and cook fish that I'd never even heard of before. Beforehand, I'd probably tried five different types of fish (including seafood): tuna, cod, mackerel, salmon, and prawns. By the time I decided to move on from this stage, I was up to double figures. This wasn't out of panic because I knew one day I wasn't going to eat fish or seafood again. But, being a bit of a geek, I was exploring the possibilities and full potential of a pescy diet for its health benefits.

While looking out for new fish to try, I did check whether it came from sustainable methods before purchasing it. I wanted to up my game and learn more about what I was eating and how it got to my plate.

Sustainable fishing methods are put in place to maintain the populations of seafood and the marine ecosystem. They guarantee that there will be populations of sea wildlife for the future. You can probably work out what the unsustainable fishing methods entail— the inevitable fast-track to extinction!

I researched what to look out for on packaging to discover whether the fish was sustainable or not:

- How the fish was raised.
- How the fish was caught.
- The inclusion of credible logos.
- Asking the person/company selling it.

If it didn't meet the criteria, I wouldn't eat the fish. However, after a while, proactively sourcing and trying new fish and seafood got a bit tedious. I'm not sure whether you'd call the taste of fish a love/hate thing, but it certainly smells more pungent than meat.

Before you even reach the eating part, you have to contend with the 'prepping', where you cook the fish and basically stink your whole household out!

Because of the smell, fish is likely to gain you (often unwanted) attention. If you're the type of person who regularly preps food and eats on the go, you'll know that eating smelly food in a public place doesn't get you many fans! This is particularly the case if you're eating in an enclosed space, such as on public transport or in a staff room.

So, if you're going pescy, you may need to adjust your food prep to avoid this. Unless, of course, you're looking to strike up an awkward conversation with someone, or annoy your family or colleagues!

"You have to eat fish because you can only get your omega 3s and 6s from them"

Omega-3 fatty acids play a crucial role in brain function, as well as normal growth and development. Well-known organisations such as the American Heart Association (AHA) recommend eating 'fatty' fish such as mackerel, sardines, herring, and salmon at least twice a week. Omega-3s have also become popular in the mainstream because they may reduce the risk of heart disease. Symptoms of omega-3 fatty acid deficiency include fatigue, poor memory, dry skin, heart problems, mood swings, depression, and poor circulation.

There are three important omega-3 fatty acids, and they can be consumed through diet or converted from one to the other in the body:

- Alphalinolenic acid (ALA): Found in a wide range of foods. It's known as a short-chain (18 carbon) omega-3 fatty acid. The human body can't make its own ALA. It must therefore be obtained through diet. (I have compiled a list of foods for your reference at the back of this section.)
- Eicosapentaenoic acid (EPA): Found mainly in fish. It's known as a long-chain (20 carbon) omega-3 fatty acid. Some EPA is converted into series 3 eicosanoids, which can reduce blood clotting, inflammation, blood pressure, and cholesterol. The human body can produce EPA out of ALA and DHA.
- Docosahexaenoic acid (DHA): Found mainly in fish and seaweed. It's known as a long-chain (22 carbon) omega-3 fatty acid and is a major component in the grey matter of the brain. It can also be found in the retina, testis, sperm, and cell membranes. The human body can convert EPA into DHA.

The main reason for this fish misconception is because it's well-known that there are virtually no 'vegan-friendly' sources of DHA or EPA (other than algae or supplements). These supplements typically come from fish and seafood, which contain both DHA and EPA. Some speciality egg and dairy products may also include them.

However, what a lot of people don't realise is that ALA consumed via plant-based foods can be converted to DHA and EPA in the body. This makes fish and seafood non-essential. In order for non-fish-eaters to get enough DHA and EPA, they must rely on their body's natural ability to make it from omega-3. This isn't just a potential issue for vegans and vegetarians though, as you'll see later in this section.

Since our bodies make DHA and EPA from omega-3, you'd naturally assume that eating lots of omega-3 foods will ensure we make enough DHA and EPA. However, it's not that simple, as research suggests that omega-6 intake inhibits the conversion of omega-3 into DHA and EPA.

Along with omega-3 fatty acids, omega-6 fatty acids play a crucial role in brain function, and normal growth and development. They're also known to stimulate skin and hair growth, maintain bone health, regulate metabolism, and maintain the reproductive system. Although there are similarities, it's important to note that omega-3 and omega-6 are not quite the same—as omega-3 fatty acids help reduce inflammation, while some omega-6 fatty acids tend to promote inflammation. With these conflicting roles, it's important to balance them out through a heathy diet.

The ideal ratio is thought to be anything between 1:1 of both and 1 omega-3 to 4 omega-6. The more even the ratio, the more the body can convert omega-3 to DHA and EPA. Some studies suggest that our ancestors would have consumed a diet closer to even.

It's important to note that if you don't get your omega-3 from fish, the efficiency of the conversion isn't great. So you may want to supplement with a vegan-friendly EPA and DHA somewhere down the line. Consuming relatively large amounts of ALA for adults is thought to convert to around 6% for EPA and 4% for DHA. Other studies suggest that between 8%-20% of ALA is converted to EPA and between 1%-9% of ALA is converted to DHA. And that's in a relatively even ratio of omega-6 to omega-3. Without an even ratio at times, the conversion wasn't even noticeable.

If you read into this area yourself, you'll see that this is why many people claim a plant-based diet is flawed. However, it goes back to the individual again—not the diet overall. Although non-fish-eaters were found to have lower levels of long chain omega-3 fatty acids (EPA and DHA) in many studies, one UK study (2010) found that vegan women on average had higher DHA levels than even the fish-eaters!

From my research, it appears that the most prevalent and important factor is having a more evenly-balanced ratio. The typical American diet tends to contain 14-25 times more omega-6 than omega-3, which could potentially be scaled down for the UK mainstream diet. What this means is that it's not just vegans and vegetarians who may not be converting enough DHA and EPA.

In fact, cardiovascular diseases and inflammatory responses have been linked to this ratio being skew-whiff (and you'll see why when we go through some examples of what popular foods could be causing this). The good news is that a more even omega-6 to omega-3 ratio can prevent or reverse these diseases. In fact, having an extreme ratio or a balanced ratio could affect humans in either a negative or positive way on a huge scale!

For example, one study found that a lower omega-6 to omega-3 ratio in women was associated with decreased risk of breast cancer, a ratio of 3:1 suppressed inflammation in patients with rheumatoid arthritis, and a ratio of 5:1 had a beneficial effect on asthmatic patients. On the other hand, a ratio of 10:1 had adverse consequences. From these findings, you can see that even working with a 1:1 ratio can have massive disease prevention benefits.

You've probably heard of the "Mediterranean diet", right? This diet is like an early "clean eating" template, because it doesn't promote processed foods and does promote more fresh, single ingredient foods. The diet became popular because studies showed that those who ate a Mediterranean diet were less likely to develop heart disease. It also has a healthier and more appropriate balance of omega-3 and omega-6 compared to the conventional Western diet.

In a nutshell, the Mediterranean diet doesn't include as much meat and processed food (which is high in omega-6) and includes more foods rich in omega-3, including whole grains, fresh fruits and vegetables, fish, olive oil, garlic, and moderate wine consumption. (The wine part may be the reason why people like to entertain this diet!).

Naturally, one of the easiest ways to reduce your omega-6 level is to reduce your animal product intake (that old chestnut again!). There are other foods you can reduce too, such as some vegetable oils. However, unless you're taking an omega-3 supplement, it's extremely difficult to get a 1:1 ratio. Even foods that are considered a good source of omega-3 may also have omega-6 in them, sometimes even more than they have omega-3!

The RDA for omega-3 intake is said to be 1.1 g per day (1100mg) for adult females and 1.6 g per day (1600mg) for adult males. This is sometimes referred to as being "adequate". These numbers fluctuate slightly, as mainstream health organisations have released their own expert opinions, and the RDA values vary considerably between countries and organisations.

There are some plant-based sources of omega-3 that can help you get a better omega balance, and we'll look at these now.

Seeds:

Flaxseeds are one of the best plant-based sources of omega-3. In 100g, there's 22810mg of omega-3, meaning a 30g serving provides 6843mg—around four times the RDA. To get an even bigger boost, you can take a tablespoon of flaxseed oil, which equates to around 7270mg of omega-3. There is some omega-6 (1940mg) in there too, but that's a huge ratio favouring omega-3.

Likewise, 30g of chia seeds delivers around 5350mg of omega-3 and just 1750mg of omega-6—a very favourable ratio! On the other hand, hemp seeds provide up to 2120mg omega-3 but 5050mg of omega-6 per 30g serving, and sesame seeds have around 6x more omega-6 than omega-3.

Nuts:

Walnuts and walnut oil are known to be a good source, however their ratio is around 5x omega-6 to omega-3. Pecans, pistachios, macadamias, cashews, peanuts, Brazil nuts, and almonds also have trace amounts of omega-3.

Vegetables:

Broccoli, Brussels sprouts, butternut squash, cauliflower, collards, kale, and spinach have an equal ratio, or a slightly more favourable omega-3 ratio.

Fruits:

Mangoes are thought to have more omega-3 than omega-6. Honeydew melons have equal amounts. Blueberries contain both, but more omega-6.

Grains:

Wild rice provides around 100mg omega-3 and around 120mg of omega-6 per 250g serving.

Beans:

Per 100g, pinto beans contain 140mg omega-3 and 100mg omega-6. Mung beans and kidney beans contain both, but the ratio favours omega-6.

Oils:

Various types of oil including soybean, mustard, rapeseed, canola, olive, and flaxseed are known to contain omega-3. But aside from flaxseed oil, the other types contain a very high amount of omega-6 compared to omega-3.

Fortified foods:

You can find foods fortified with omega-3 such as some tofu, bread, juice, energy bars, margarine/butter, and oil. However, check whether it has been added by way of fish oil if you don't want to consume fish.

Supplements:

Omega-3 supplements are widely available, and the most popular plant-based version is flaxseed oil or flaxseed capsules. There are also omega-3 soft gels made from algae. Obviously, you can get fish oils if you're still eating fish, but in the long-term you may want to find a non-fish alternative.

You're probably thinking right now that you should reduce your omega-6 intake to get a more balanced ratio. Here are some foods known to be very rich in omega-6. Some of these you may be consuming on a regular basis or already be abstaining from, and some also appeared in our omega-3 list:

Oils:

Safflower, grape seed, sunflower, corn, wheatgerm, soybean.

Salad dressings:

French, Caesar, sesame seed, honey mustard, Italian, thousand island, mayonnaise, light mayonnaise.

Nuts and seeds:

Walnuts, pine nuts, brazil nuts, pecans, peanuts, almonds, and sesame, sunflower, and pumpkin seeds.

Snacks and fast food:

Chips, crisps, cookies, brownies, puff pastry, cake, muffins, shortbread, and deep fat fried foods including onion rings, hash browns, and chicken nuggets.

Meat and animal products:

Sausage, ham, bacon, salami, other pork cuts, chicken thigh, turkey bacon, turkey mince, chicken wings with skin, turkey meat with skin, beef ribs, lamb, eggs, milk, butter, processed cheese, and cheese varieties including cheddar, parmesan, and cream cheese.

You may have noticed there are more "junk foods" on the omega-6 list than the omega-3 list. This is often due to the oil involved in cooking these foods. For example, deep fat fried foods such as chips and mass-produced products such as cookies include some form of oil.

It appears that avoiding processed and junk foods is a great way to reduce your omega-6 intake. You can imagine why the omega-3 to omega 6 ratio in the conventional Western diet isn't great—as oils are in many mass-produced, processed, or fried foods—things that are always fun and popular!

While you transition from meat, you may well increase your consumption of nuts and seeds, which often have a high ratio of omega-6 to omega-3. However, chia seeds and flaxseed are much higher in omega-3, so it's a good idea to consume these daily. This will also account for your omega-3 intake if you exclude fish from your diet moving forward.

Body shape started changing people started commenting on it

I'll never forget a comment made by one of my clients around this time: "You look sickeningly healthy!"

As my nutrition became on point, people started to really notice that I was looking "different". More specifically, looking healthier. My theory is that the way I was feeling on the inside reflected in how I was looking on the outside. Tip top. People started telling me I was "glowing", which made me feel like I was a pregnant woman. Don't laugh.

With such a sudden change to my diet and overall lifestyle, I'd always known that a change to my physique was imminent. My initial concern was that it would be a negative change, however I knew this was in my control, and would only happen if I didn't take proper care of my nutrition along the way. Now, it had become clear that my diet was having a positive impact on my wellbeing. At the time, I had cut out meat, was eating fish once a day for dinner, drinking green smoothies in the mornings, and consuming a wide variety of plant-based food throughout the day, such as steamed vegetables.

My routine before starting this journey was very different. Not just due to the volume of meat consumption, but my priorities, the amount of training I was doing, and the calories required to support my energy levels and recovery. When I decided to write the book and put my training partially on hold, I weighed 95kg and my body fat percentage was around 12% (going by the scales I was using to measure progress throughout). I was very comfortable with this and found it easy to decrease my body fat if I wanted to. I was doing weight training 5-6 times per week, coaching 1-1, and holding group exercise classes such as indoor cycling and kettlebells.

The first noticeable thing after reducing my meat intake was losing weight. I'd lost 7kg without even realising, and my weight was comfortable at 88kg. I hadn't lost muscle, but I had started to lose some of the 'bulk', which to some people is what I was known for. Fortunately, I still felt as strong.

This is a very subjective statement, but many people said I "looked better for it" because I had been "too pumped up" before. Others said they preferred the way I looked before. Whatever anyone said, I didn't let it get to me. To people who strive for body composition like I had previously, losing weight or muscle is a travesty, as you work so hard for it over such a long time and yet you can 'lose it' so easily and quickly. Ultimately, whether or not you see it as a travesty is relative to your goals and lifestyle at the time. And I was playing the long game.

"I want to stop eating meat and fish, but I can't because I don't want to get skinny"

When it comes to a change in our diet or nutrition, a common concern is how it will affect our physical appearance. This can depend on personal preference and the times we live in. At the moment, there is a trend for women to be 'curvy' and show body-confidence, for example, in being plus-sized. A decade or so ago, it was 'trendy' to be extremely skinny.

Generally, when most people say they don't want to get "skinny", what they mean is superficially skinny, not an extreme version of malnutrition, which severely affects someone's health. Likewise, when people say "curvy", they usually don't mean an extreme version of obesity and its associated health risks.

Looks aside, there is a more serious issue that being too skinny could actually be unhealthy. People can become "too skinny" when they aren't eating enough calories to maintain their current weight. This can cause health complications down the line, as it may mean the body isn't getting enough nutrients to function optimally. This is why people associate a vegan diet with immediately getting skinny, because they aren't consuming enough calories from other foods since they stopped eating meat. As we covered earlier, it's vital to replace the calories from meat with something else. In doing so, you won't become the unhealthy kind of skinny—the malnourished kind.

There is also a reason why vegans sometimes look superficially "skinner" than meat eaters. What if I told you that eating meat and fish could be causing water retention and inflammation in your body? Forcing you to look puffy? Or puffier than you really should be? It's all about how the body uses water.

Up to 60% of the human adult body is water, and the body uses a complex system of hormones and hormone-like substances called prostaglandins to keep its volume of fluid at a constant level. Say you were to intake an excessive amount of fluid in one day, the amount of fluid would not be affected in the long term. This is because the kidneys would quickly excrete the excess fluid in the form of urine. Likewise, if you didn't get enough to drink, the body would hold on to the fluids and urinate less than usual.

However, imbalances in this system can lead to water retention, ranging from mild and unnoticeable to symptomatic, with swelling. To understand how and why this happens, we need a quick science lesson.

To work properly, the body needs sodium. It uses sodium to control blood pressure and blood volume, and for your muscles and nerves to function correctly. Most people will likely get enough without even trying. In fact, some people should be proactively looking to cut back on their sodium intake, because too much is bad for us. The RDA for sodium is 2300mg. For those with high blood pressure, it's no more than 1500mg daily.

When people hear "sodium", they often think of salt. Salt contains sodium, but they aren't the same thing. Salt (table salt) is sodium chloride: 40% sodium, 60% chloride. The average daily intake of salt in the UK is 3200mg. 1tsp of salt is said to contain 2325mg sodium, and is therefore over the recommended 'safe' amount.

Even if you have a "salty tooth", it's worth noting that having too much sodium in the diet is associated with high blood pressure in some people, which increases the risk of sudden death from heart attack or stroke.

When we consume sodium, our body releases water to excrete the sodium out in our urine, but we are left with less water, so we get thirsty and have to drink more to rebalance. This is why it's said that pubs sell salty food such as peanuts and crisps, because they make you thirsty so you order more drinks!

Sodium and water work together. When you consume sodium, the body holds on to water to keep its ideal concentration. It's thought that for every 400mg of sodium you consume, the body compensates by retaining around 1 litre of water. This could equate to excess weight through water retention of around 1kg. The average American consumes 3400mg of sodium per day, so their body will be holding around 8 litres of water, which is about an extra 8kg.

When we consume salt, water moves from the blood stream to the skin tissue, which can create a 'puffy' look. It's thought that the more you consume in a short space of time, the more noticeable the puffy look. Think back when you had a Chinese takeaway and woke up feeling dry, puffy, and bloated!

In theory, when you adopt a plant-based diet or start to abstain from certain foods that are notoriously high in sodium (such as meat and fish), then naturally you'll consume less sodium and therefore won't hold as much water.

Meat, fish, and animal products are generally considered to be high in sodium, especially in comparison to most plant-based foods. Here are some popular examples and their sodium content (per 100g):

- Milk: 43mg.
- Beef mince: 67mg.
- Egg boiled: 124mg.
- Chicken breast: 62mg.
- Bacon, fried: 1684mg.
- Cheddar cheese: 644mg.
- Salmon: 56mg.
- Mackerel: 379mg.
- Tuna, canned: 50mg.
- Cod: 78mg.
- Prawns: 111mg.

There are a few plant-based foods that contain relatively surprising levels of sodium (per 100g):

- Celery: 80mg.
- Beetroot: 78mg.
- Artichoke: 94mg.
- Carrot: 69mg.
- Turnip: 67mg.

This is how sodium levels are considered:

- High sodium: Foods that contain more than 400mg per serving.
- Moderate sodium: Foods that contain between 140mg-400mg.
- Low sodium: Foods that have 140mg or less in one serving.
- Very low sodium: Foods that have 35mg or less per serving.
- Sodium-free: Foods that have less than 5mg per serving.

You can rest assured that most plant-based food will be low in sodium, with the exception of plant-based products. This includes things like sauces (for example, soy sauce is notoriously high in sodium), canned foods (beans, fruit, and vegetables), cereals, nuts (salted and roasted), and dressings. This excess will usually be in the form of added salt.

Talking openly about being a pescatarian

Once people had started to notice my body shape changing, they became curious how I had achieved this, and it became harder to not let on. People would ask me questions about my private life, my diet, my training, my reasons for the change, etc. This was especially difficult as I never lie about anything! And I just got fed up with not being myself in conversation.

When I openly admitted that I was eating a pescatarian diet and had been for some time, I felt relieved. Contrary to what I thought would happen, most people were intrigued, and not once did they question my motives. Nobody questioned why I didn't eat meat, or whether I was heading for a vegetarian or vegan diet. In fact, the majority applauded me for it and said things like:

"I wish I ate more fish!"
"Fish is really healthy for you!"
"I would like to try that sometime!"
"Good for you!"

And my personal favourite,
"Isn't that a vegetarian who eats fish?"

Unlike the negative vibes I'd heard about in response to the "extreme" vegan diet, the pescy diet got a big thumbs up, going by the people I spoke to. What seemed consistent from all of the reactions was fish = protein. Protein = good. Fish = better for you than meat. Meat = bad for you. Interestingly, the majority of these people ate more meat than fish.

Not once did I suggest that others should follow suit and try to emulate my diet. However, some of my clients did this without telling me and attempted their own version of a pescy diet or replacing more meat with fish. After talking about it briefly, they said things like, I had inspired them, they "wanted to give it a go" as it had worked for me, and that they "enjoyed it more anyway". A couple of them even tried tofu in place of meat. However, some weren't sure whether it was good for them, having heard mixed reviews, and wanted my opinion.

The experience taught me that some people had been thinking about trying this for a while, and they could make the change fairly easily because they wanted to swap meat for fish. I believed they would be more likely to see it through if they had a positive influence, someone who would support them.

"You shouldn't eat tofu and soya because they can lower testosterone, mess with oestrogen levels, and can give men boobs"

"If you swallow bubble gum, it'll take seven years to digest."
"If you pull a funny face and the wind changes, you'll get stuck like that."
"If you say Beetlejuice three times, he will appear."

Do you remember these sayings as a kid? They're very memorable, and we were very impressionable. As adults, we should know better, but let's face it, it's a lot easier to take them as truth than to do the research yourself. In the case of this misconception, if someone brings up hormones, then you know looking into it yourself is going to be long-winded. So, you'd probably rather believe it must be scientifically proven to save you the effort.

The soybean is recognised as a good plant-based source of protein as an alternative to animal products, because it contains all of the essential amino acids, as well as vitamins and minerals. The composition of these nutrients varies among preparations, but it is in the highest quantity in whole soy foods such as edamame (whole soy beans), soy milk, tofu, and tempeh. Some of the minerals in soy include calcium, iron, magnesium, manganese, phosphorus, potassium, and zinc. It also contains many B vitamins and vitamin C, as well as fibre, omega-3, and omega-6 fatty acids. Sounds good, right? So what's the deal with soy and the whole man boobs ("moobs") thing?

Gynecomastia is the medical term for developed breasts in men, which is what some people insinuate will happen to men if they eat soy. If this was true, there would be a lot of men in need of bras! Particularly in eastern and south east Asia, where soy is a staple in both men's and women's diets.

Soy protein consumption per person is reported to be less than 1g per day in most European and North American countries, including the UK and U.S. In Japan, average consumption is 8.7g of soy protein per day; in Korea, 6.2–9.6g; Indonesia, 7.4g; and China, 3.4g.

If you care to question someone who proclaims that soy gives you "moobs" they'll usually point to 'hormones' or mention 'isoflavones' and/or 'oestrogen'. However, studies in men show that isoflavones do not affect testosterone levels or circulating oestrogen levels. Even for isoflavone levels that are significantly higher than a typical Asian male consuming a soy-rich diet, there is no evidence of feminizing effects.

It's believed that the "soy causes man boobs" myth is rooted in the confusion between oestrogen and phytoestrogen. Isoflavones are a type of naturally occurring isoflavonoids, many of which act as phytoestrogens in mammals. Phytoestrogen is not oestrogen. However, phytoestrogens are naturally-occurring plant compounds that are structurally and/or functionally similar to oestrogen and their active substances. Oestrogen and testosterone are steroid hormones that occur naturally in both sexes and animals used for food.

The ironic thing is that nobody ever brings up how meat, dairy, and eggs all contain phytoestrogens too, because these animals consume plant foods! By avoiding soy, you are not avoiding phytoestrogens.

The subject of soy hasn't only been debated in the context of male hormones. Controversy and debate has also surrounded its effect on female sex hormones too. The conclusions of these studies go back and forth, and outcomes vary depending on what is being tested.

If you're interested, I suggest you look into this area yourself. You can check my references, do some research, and make your own call on soy consumption in your diet. Having weighed it up over a fair amount of research, my personal belief is that soy is safe to consume and non-conflicting hormonally. That is, provided the source is non-GMO soybean, eaten in moderation, and included as part of a nutritious, varied plant-based diet.

GMO stands for 'genetically modified organism' and is defined to be: Any organism whose genetic material has been altered using genetic engineering techniques (i.e. a genetically engineered organism).

Similar to the section on toxins, I'm not going to take things too deep here, as I don't want this book to turn into a science degree! What I will say is that GMOs have become a controversial subject in their usage in food for both humans and animals, to the point where it almost crosses the line into conspiracy theories.

Having done a fair amount of research into GMOs, I personally would never consume something that wasn't 'non-GMO' unless I had no idea I was consuming it, or was completely desperate i.e. to avoid actual starvation! If you want to find out more on this subject, there are some documentaries I'd recommend at the back of the book.

Meat and fish = an expensive habit

From an economic standpoint, I hadn't worked out whether it was cheaper to be a pescy or a classic meat eater yet. So I decided to put it to the test. The next time I went to the supermarket for my weekly shop, I checked out my receipt. It was clear where the majority of the expenditure came from: the bloody fish! It was also clear what the cheapest foods were: the veggies!

I used to spend up to £50 a week on meat, fish, and animal products alone. Not to mention supplements such as whey protein and bars. Of course, I have to factor in spending more money on fruit, vegetables, grains, nuts, seeds, and beans now, but my weekly shop is around £30-£40 cheaper per week than back then! By dropping meat and fish, I save around £160 a month!

The economic thing got to me a bit and I started tallying up the benefits of a plant-based diet, and including more vegetables. At the time, the specific protein sources I was eating were eggs, cheese, whey protein, salmon, cod, tuna, prawns, nuts, nut butters, seeds, and tofu. I wasn't aware of the other plant-based sources of protein available to me. So I weighed up my options moving forward, knowing that I wouldn't be entirely confident moving to the next stage just yet:

1. Eat more of the same protein sources I was already eating, other than animal products.
2. Research more plant-based proteins and implement them into my diet now.
3. Keep going as I am, because I feel good.

I went with option three, because it felt like the most 'natural' thing to do at that point.

"I don't want to eat more vegetables because they go straight through me"

Right, it's time to talk bathroom habits. The average person does a number two once a day and the "normal" range is reported to be anywhere between once every three days to three times per day. It's also reported that the average person lets go of around 30g of waste per 5-6kg of body weight. That means a person weighing around 70kg will lose around half a kg each day, and you can adjust this depending on weight.

Going any more than four times per day, and producing watery, loose stools could be classified as diarrhoea. This can be triggered by infections, medication, Irritable Bowel Syndrome (IBS), and diet (the classic "it must be something that I ate").

IBS is a common, long-term condition that affects the digestive system. It can cause bouts of stomach cramps, bloating, diarrhoea, and/or constipation, because food passes through your gut too slowly or too quickly. IBS is thought to affect up to 1 in 5 people at some point in their life, and usually first appears between 20 and 30 years of age. Around twice as many women are affected by IBS as men.

You may suffer with IBS or know someone who does. Either way, it's a reason why something might pass right through you. The symptoms vary between individuals and affect some people more severely than others. Symptoms tend to come and go in periods that last from a few days to a few months, often during times of stress or after eating certain foods. The exact cause of IBS is unknown, but most experts believe it's related to increased sensitivity of the gut and problems digesting food. Ways to prevent IBS include:

- Identify and avoid foods that trigger your symptoms.
- Alter the amount of fibre in your diet.
- Get more exercise.
- Reduce stress levels.

When it comes to diet and eating more veggies, your bathroom habits may change. Prior to my plant-based diet, I had less frequent and more inconsistent number 2s than I do now. Nothing majorly bad, in the "normal" range, no IBS, no constipation, and rarely diarrhoea. However, my bathroom schedule would vary in terms of timing. Nowadays, my number 2s are very frequent, but still in the "normal" range. The end result is super consistent too. Often, the "ideal". Plus, it's always over double-quick.

Going to the toilet could be considered perfectly healthy, and eating more veggies may be even lead to an improvement in your digestive health. Provided you are in the "normal" range (up to three times per day), and whether or not you have been diagnosed with IBS, going slightly more, or quicker, generally isn't anything to worry about.

Jumping the veggie gun

I realised that if I wanted to nail this and reach the veggie stage, I should probably stop buying fish. I mean, this was the only way fish was getting into my house!

So while I phased it out, I purchased more eggs to swap for fish at dinner time. As I rotated my meals for the days ahead, I would potentially be eating eggs twice a day, morning and night. Going by my greedy portions, that was up to 10+ whole eggs a day! Styles included omelettes, boiled, scrambled, poached, and fried. After a week of trying this out:

- I missed fish in the evening.
- I felt unhealthier in myself.
- I was bored of eggs.

All in all, I didn't feel ready to make the adjustment to the next stage. I probably could have persisted with this new routine, but it would have completely broken my 'natural' rule, which seemed to be working wonders up to this point—as I felt top notch! I knew that if I wanted to achieve my goal of moving on to the next stage, I would have to phase out fish at some point. But when the following week rolled around, I bought salmon and started eating it in the evenings again! I felt like I had to.

Looking back, what I ultimately needed was to create more variety with food that wasn't fish. I failed to move forward on my first attempt because I depended too much on old habits and kept my meal prep too rigid just to suit the "P word" (protein).

"Fish is better for you than meat"

Fish have a higher proportion of omega-3s and "healthy fats" than meat, and this is often the topic of the mainstream debate over why fish may be better for you than meat. These so-called "healthy fats" are monounsaturated and polyunsaturated fats, and they are known to improve blood cholesterol levels and lower the risk of heart disease.

Plant-based sources of monounsaturated fat:

Avocados, almonds, peanuts, cashews, Brazil nuts, hazelnuts, macadamia nuts, pecans, and pistachios. Nut butters such as peanut, almond, and cashew. Oils such as olive, canola, peanut, safflower, and sesame.

Plant-based sources of polyunsaturated fat:

Oils such as rapeseed, soybean, corn, and sunflower. Some nuts and seeds such as walnuts, pecans, pistachios, pine nuts, chia, sesame, pumpkin and sunflower. Tofu, tahini, soybeans, and flaxseed.

Saturated fat content can be high in meat, especially processed meat, and other animal products such as milk and cheese. It's thought that by substituting saturated fat in your diet for monounsaturated and polyunsaturated fats, you may be able to keep your HDL (good) cholesterol levels high and your LDL (bad) cholesterol levels low.

The current RDA for total fat is 70g in the UK, based on a total daily calorie intake of 2000kcal. Although there aren't specific recommendations for unsaturated fat intake, it's recommended that healthy fats make up the majority of your total fat. Provided that your total fat intake is in line with your nutritional requirements, it's thought that the more unsaturated fats, the better.

To reduce your saturated fat intake, opt for leaner types of meat, animal products, fish, and seafood (if you haven't stopped eating them already). You can also utilise "healthier" cooking methods, such as grilling, baking, boiling, or poaching rather than frying. Avoid foods that are battered, fried, or sautéed in a lot of oil.

You can also switch products high in saturated fats, such as mayonnaise or dressings, with those high in monounsaturated and polyunsaturated fats, such as avocados, nuts, and olive oil. Especially if you want to jazz up a salad.

So, is fish better for you than meat? Going by its saturated fat content, you could say that. However, when eaten in abundance, fish is thought to potentially cause long-term harm in poisoning through toxins and chemicals such as mercury. For example, pregnant and breastfeeding women are advised to carefully measure their fish intake and not eat fish with high mercury content, as it can harm their baby. They're also advised not to eat more than two portions of oily fish per week and to avoid shellfish altogether. Children are often advised similarly, and guidelines differ according to age.

If I could go back and do anything different at this stage, I would at least have gone for fish that had the lowest amounts of mercury. In order of least to most mercury, these are: mussels, squid, Atlantic mackerel, salmon, cod, lobster, haddock, skipjack tuna, Spanish mackerel, bluefin tuna, swordfish.

Debating whether this is the end

For me, the pescy stage was the most memorable on my journey. Although I knew I was "kind of healthy" before starting all of this, I genuinely felt healthier now. It truly felt like the upgrade to my previous lifestyle. I knew more about nutrition than ever before, and was feeling good about pretty much everything!

The downside is I was seriously debating whether I should keep moving forward towards a plant-based diet, because I couldn't guarantee I would still be feeling this good! Especially because I'd already tried to stop eating fish and gone a week before reverting to old habits, as I didn't feel that good. Weirdly, my gut feeling was that there was more to all of this. Something seemed too good to be true.

I'd already touched on the health and economic aspects of eliminating fish, but in terms of motivation, the message just wasn't sinking in. Ethically, I still wasn't up to the same standard as land animals. And due to my recent comforts, I'd become sloppy on the back end of the journey—the research. There turned out to be many documentaries that shed light on why someone would want to progress toward a plant-based diet. Of those, there was one documentary that many threads and comments pointed towards: Earthlings.

The comments made it clear that Earthlings was a major instigator for some people switching to a plant-based diet and actually sticking to it! This was promising—just what I needed to move to the next stage. However, I was a bit sceptical, as it didn't sound like my cup of tea. The opposite in fact! Comments said that Earthlings was "very deep", "gory", and "hard to watch". It contained a lot of footage of animals being slaughtered and made the slaughterhouse workers look like murderers from the horror film Hostel. I like to keep things chirpy and educational, but it sounded like this was going to shock my system. So I procrastinated a while. "The truth hurts," as they say.

One evening, I braced myself and watched it start to finish. I didn't cry, but I did feel very sad and ashamed at the way animals of land and sea are treated by humans in this day and age. It's difficult to know what I mean unless you watch it for yourself—but only do so if you have a strong stomach. You don't have to watch the documentary to transition to a plant-based diet, but it's one of the reasons I was able to move on from the pescy stage being assured that I was on the right road.

"I already know that animals and fish have to be killed for me to eat them, so why does this fact have to be rammed down my throat? Isn't it 'normal' to eat animals anyway?"

This is a common thing you might hear, and to anyone who thinks this way, there are questions they should ask themselves before trying to justify why they don't want to watch or learn where their food comes from:

- If you can't bring yourself to watch where your food comes from, then should you really be putting it in your body?
- If it's not good enough for your eyes—is it good enough for your stomach?
- If you can't bring yourself to learn anything about the process in further detail, isn't something telling you this might not be as "natural" or "normal" as you might think?

These questions aren't directed at you personally—they're just questions that someone may want to consider. If this conversation ever arose with someone, you don't have to be the one who asks these questions.

The ethical side of the process often brings up the most heated reactions and is a real emotional hotspot surrounding the vegan topic. Many people have already justified to themselves why they need to eat animals. And you'll be in the process of trying to understand why you've justified to your-self that you don't need to eat them.

Unless someone has the desire to further their knowledge on where their food came from, they will likely be happy to keep going as they are. To them, the thought of learning something new that could ignite change in routine may make them feel uncomfortable and protective of their current beliefs.

Fish have feelings too

Spoiler alert! Watching the unjust suffering of so many fish in Earthlings really caught my attention. Seeing them being pulled out of the water by the truckload and being left to suffocate or have their throats slit was absurd viewing. It was on a level that I hadn't seen before. And it was clear from the documentary that they absolutely do feel pain and suffering in the same way that land animals do. Morally, I got the feeling of wrong-doing.

As well as realising there was no logic or consistency in why land animals are considered more important than those in the sea, I also discovered from the documentary that there's a name for unfair favouritism against animals: "speciesism". It's defined as: The assumption of human superiority leading to the exploitation of animals. This applies to all types of animals.

Deep down, I always knew that seeing where my meat and fish came from would affect my relationship with food, and therefore my protein intake. I knew it would take me out of my comfort zone and question my morals. That it would lead to change. So, I did my best to avoid this for a while.

Earthlings showed that although the general public like to think there is a "humane" way of killing an animal, there really isn't. In fact, the word "humane" had become a popular term used by animal eaters to justify where their meat, fish, and animal products came from, and how they were slaughtered. They knew something had died or been extorted, but believed it was done in the best possible way, where the animal had never suffered. However, although they believed this to be the case, they hadn't actually researched it to find out the truth. I'd definitely been one of those people up to this point.

I checked out synonyms for the word "slaughter", which is the most common word used to reflect the outcome of killing animals, and the list shocked me: annihilate, assassinate, bloodbath, bloodshed, butchery, carnage, decimation, destroy, drown, eliminate, execute, genocide, hit, holocaust, homicide kill off, liquidate, massacre, mow down, murder, poison, put to death, slay, wipe out... I didn't want to be associated with any of that!

"Animals don't feel pain like humans do, and fish don't feel pain"

Something that all animals (including fish) and humans have in common is their sentient status (sentience). This is defined as: The ability to perceive or feel things.

When you look further into this, it means that animals have more similarities to humans and are more advanced than we give them credit for. They pretty much share the same needs and desires for adaptation and survival as humans do. Examples of these necessities and similarities include:

- Food and water.
- Shelter and companionship.
- Freedom of movement.
- Avoidance of pain.

Animals naturally do their best to live for pleasure and to avoid painful experiences. Physically and psychologically, they can feel, and what's more, they can remember these experiences. They are therefore motivated by both pain and pleasure. They are hedonistic. Does this sound familiar to any other species? Us for example? And how would we know that they don't feel these experiences in a more extreme way than humans?

Both humans and animals inhabit a nervous system. This is the network of nerve cells and fibres that transmit nerve impulses between parts of the body. It's ultimately what is responsible for whether a living thing (such as humans and animals) feels pain or not. Without a nervous system, a living being wouldn't feel pain, so this is a big indicator whether something could be considered a "sentient being" or not. I'm not just talking about physical pain here, like stubbing your toe, but also psychological pain like a crappy day at work, or an upsetting break-up.

To understand how an animal attempts to avoid painful experiences, both emotional or physical, think about a rescue dog's demeanour, be it timid, aggressive, or unpredictable. Likewise, this isn't just be the case for dogs, as all animals can feel this way provided they have a nervous system that registers pain. ·

Even fish demonstrate high levels of stress if they are removed from their natural habitat, the water. In most cases, they are seen to make violent attempts to escape the clutches of humans, other animals, or machinery by flapping around and even biting. This clearly shows some sort of reaction to pain or avoidance to pain, even in their own fishy way.

Fish finger Fridays and phasing out fish

With my new-found desire and motivation to stop eating fish (or you could say "flesh") altogether, I'd finally made up my mind to progress to the next stage. No longer would my diet be that of a "vegetarian who eats fish".

From previous experience and research, I identified that suddenly going down the abolish route may not be the best way for me to retain the change long term. In fact, it may increase the chances of a bounce-back! So, I decided to gradually phase it out until I no longer "needed" it in my routine.

As I was only eating fish and seafood in the evenings, my gut feeling said the most obvious route was to reduce the number of evenings I ate it from 6-7 per week, halving my intake each week, until it was 0 evenings per week:

- Week 1 = 3-4 times per week.
- Week 2 = 2-3 times per week.
- Week 3 = 1-2 times per week.
- Week 4 = 0-1 times per week.

This was the first time frame I had given myself throughout the whole process, as I had always gone with what felt natural. But it turned out that through watching Earthlings and doing more associated research, I very naturally and quickly shot to week 4. Essentially, it made my plan a waste of time, as I didn't fancy eating fish anymore. Well, except on Fridays that is!

On Fridays, I would have a relaxing night in, with fish fingers and steamed vegetables (spinach, corn on the cob, peas) for dinner. It was nice to keep things low-maintenance, familiar, cheap, and cheerful after a long week. Believe it or not, as tacky a habit as it sounds, it was actually an "upgrade" from the previous cod, chips, and mushy peas from the fish and chip shop. The new habit wasn't as tasty, but it at least felt healthier than a takeaway!

Before week 4 was up, I was able to not eat fish. I had no desire to eat it whatsoever—and was ready to switch to a completely vegetarian diet. Yet "fish finger Fridays" stayed around for a few weeks. Looking back, I think it was because frozen fish fingers don't look or taste anything like fish or flesh. Besides, I couldn't think of another catchy name for my Friday night theme!

"You'd have to hunt and eat animals/ fish if you were stranded on a desert island, and an animal would eat you if it had the chance"

What we have here is a fantasy. One that tries to paint a plant-based diet as inconvenient and unsustainable. A fantasy made up to present a "do or die" scenario that is very unlikely to ever happen. Unless you plan on applying for Bear Grylls The Island or another of those TV shows.

The answer these people need to hear from you is: "Yes I would." From experience, if you don't give them this answer instantaneously, the fantasy will escalate to become even more unrealistic and impossible. All with the intention of trying to coerce you into saying you would still eat animals.

"What if there was no other food but fish?"
"What if you were going to die the next day if you didn't?"
"What if the animal was going to kill you first?"

In this situation, you can keep your true thoughts to yourself and deflect from the conversation by saying something like: "That would never happen." And you can change the subject if you don't want to be drawn into a debate. I've also had some joy with this before. If I'm in a funny mood, I escalate things myself and turn it around: "Would you turn vegan if you were stranded on a desert island and all you had to live off was plant-based food?" Half the time I don't get an answer. I have a feeling the answer would be yes though!

You could play the "what if" game all day long with someone if you wanted to. But unless you're having fun and turning it into a bit of banter like I try to, what good will come of it? You'll never really know "what if" unless you actually find yourself in that situation, which is not likely so there's no point preparing for it. Even in your own head. If an animal was attempting to eat you, the best defence might not be to attempt to eat it back during the scuffle!

I have a lot of thoughts about humans as a survival species. I wouldn't ever discredit the need for survival or adaptation. Past, present, and future. I mean, we have got this far haven't we? However, I live just outside London, and I've never met anyone who had to hunt animals of any kind to survive around here. I've also not heard of many incidences in my local area where someone had to eat an animal before it ate them first!

PESCATARIAN summary

Be patient—slow and steady wins the race.

Do what you feel is right, when you feel it's right to do so. If you want to try new foods, then go for it. If the food you want to try is suitable for that stage, then it should be "guilt-free" until you decide that it's not suitable. For example, fish.

Identify recipes that you will enjoy and stick to them.

While you begin to trial new foods, you may be stuck in your old ways of cooking. Look to recipe books that suit your nutritional requirements and tastes for new-found inspiration and knowledge.

Take note of any changes to your health.

Your actions, good or bad, will have a positive or negative effect on your health at some point. The start of any new diet will always be a bit of trial and error. By noting any changes, you are tracking what's best for you.

Buy and use a steamer.

Experiment with new combinations of veggies and steam them all at once. If possible, prep your veggies at home for convenience and keep them with you in some Tupperware so you can eat on the go. You'll be more likely to eat them, because you won't want to waste them!

Drink more smoothies.

Why not attempt to make this part of your new morning routine (where possible)? Experiment with smoothie recipes if you're looking for some inspiration. Green-based smoothies are a popular choice in the mainstream to keep the nutrients high and the calories and sugar low.

Look at your food shopping receipts.

Look at the single highest-priced items. If it's meat, fish, or animal products and you think that it's expensive, look into plant-based alternatives that are nutritionally similar and cheaper overall.

Don't be scared to poo.

If you're apprehensive about going to toilet more due to consuming additional fibre in plant-based foods, then don't be! As long as your stools are healthy and regular, then this is perfectly healthy. You'll get used to it.

Watch more related documentaries and learn more.

People take in information in many different ways. The four main ways are: visual, audio, verbal, and physical. Documentaries promote two of the four. If documentaries aren't for you, try other methods to learn more. There's more information on documentaries I recommend in the What now? section at the back of the book.

Keep it as real as possible.

It's great to have a guideline, for example, a diet plan. However, planning ahead in too much detail can cause unnecessary pressure on your journey. You're not a robot, so take into account the many variables of life.

Stage Three
VEGETARIAN

Being a vegetarian is actually really easy

Definition of a vegetarian: A person who does not eat meat or fish, and sometimes other animal products, especially for moral, religious, or health reasons.

Although this definition makes the veggie diet out to be somewhat restrictive, sourcing suitable foods at this stage was easier than it had been before.

It turned out that many mainstream supermarkets and high street restaurants accommodated for those on a vegetarian diet by offering alternative choices and highlighting the options as veggie-friendly. Further information on the menu showed that some main dishes could be altered to suit dietary requirements, and all you had to do was ask the waiter or chef! Never before had I noticed how prominent an all-out vegetarian diet was in society. It felt good to know that even people with little knowledge of nutrition could easily identify whether something was suitable for them or not.

I went to a traditional, old school English cafe for breakfast and even they had a vegetarian menu! Before seeing the menu, my gut feeling was that I'd have to build my own meal from whatever they had available, and it would cost more because it would be too "fancy" for them to handle. Turns out that an omelette and salad isn't that fancy after all—I was clearly overthinking it!

Although it seemed convenient in everyday life, I was also a little apprehensive about the diet's potential health benefits in the early stages because:

- My options were becoming more and more limited.
- My knowledge of plant-based proteins had not progressed much since the beginning.
- I'd tried a vegetarian diet briefly before and it didn't go so well. Whoops.

As well as seeing a vegetarian section on menus, I noticed a vegetarian frozen section in the supermarket and a vegetarian hallmark on snack foods. It seemed that a veggie certainly wouldn't go hungry, even if the nutritional options weren't always up to scratch!

"Eggs are good for you. Eggs are bad for you. Who knows? Let's eat them anyway"

I was born in 1988, and my first take on the subject, at around 5 years old, was that eggs were really bad for you. This was on the basis that they have "high cholesterol content". Of course, back then, I had no idea what this meant. But as far as I could gather, you shouldn't eat a lot of them!

Fast forward to 2004 and I was still upholding this belief... That was until some information surfaced in the mainstream about egg whites being good for you and egg yolks being bad for you. Here the confusion began! I was gutted. The yolk was my favourite part. When eating a fried egg, I used to purposely (and carefully) eat the yolk all in one mouthful. It was tradition.

Now I was having to rethink that procedure because egg yolks were well-known in the mainstream to be detrimental to our health. Something about "heart disease", which is what the whole "cholesterol" thing was about. That, and the yolk was supposedly the only part of the egg that contained fat.

The egg white was supposedly all protein and the most "bioavailable" part. I also had no idea what "bioavailable" meant, but classically went along with it because it sounded sciency and therefore too longwinded to get into! For reference, as I learnt, bioavailability has many definitions, but in this context, it refers to how well something is absorbed.

During my late teens, I got more interested in nutrition (as well as a shitload of partying!). I started to train with weights for body composition and image, rather than just for exercise and to keep active. This tied into a thought-out increase in protein, which led to greater egg white consumption. The theory was egg whites = protein. Protein = muscle. More protein = more muscle.

The yolk continued to go in the bin. Or to a friend, relative, or whoever would save it if they happened to be around before it went in the bin! Egg yolk = fat. Fat = more body fat.

I took note as products began to infiltrate the mainstream—capitalising on the widespread word that egg whites do nothing but good. You could now buy liquid egg whites, saving so much aggro! If you've ever tried to dissect an egg white from the yolk without knowing the most efficient technique, you'll know where I'm coming from! It's messy and tedious (without swearing).

Fast forward to 2013, I was 25. The mainstream agenda on eggs turned to the yolk now being good for you! Low carb, high fat, and "clean eating" was in. Whole eggs fit the bill if you were following this diet, because the mainstream belief was that eggs are a "clean" food. The whole egg was also now believed to contain nutrients that may lower the risk of heart disease, including protein, and vitamins B2, B9, B12, and D.

This was a total contradiction of past mainstream media information. For the first time, I decided to experiment with this in my own diet. I soon realised I couldn't eat as many eggs in a single sitting as before. Roughly around half the amount, evidently due to the calories in a whole egg being more filling. A whole egg is 155 kcal per 100g, while egg whites are 52 kcal per 100g.

Given that I was eating as much "clean fat" as possible, I thought this was so much better. Provided it came from a "natural" source such as meat, fish, or animal products of course. It was less fiddly and cheaper than the egg white scenario. It also felt more natural, like an all-or-nothing approach to eggs. I stuck with this belief all the way up to my transition to a plant-based diet and I was quite fond of omelettes the whole way through!

In the end, what did it for me was the simple reality that there's no solid, overwhelming evidence that proves whether eggs are good for you or not. Some evidence suggests they're a "superfood". Other research led my gut feeling to say they're more likely bad for you. Mainly because, unlike all plant foods, all animal products contain cholesterol, which is one of the leading causes of atherosclerosis (we'll go into this later in the book).

Suddenly, everyone's a veggie!

Some studies suggest that vegetarians make up between 7-11% of the UK adult population, which is around 4 million people (and rising). Although many people believe this diet simply means you don't eat meat, there is a level of understanding from non-veggies. In the mainstream, people seem to "get it" and aren't not too judgemental of it.

When I took more interest in the veggie diet, I started to have conversations with people about it and realised just how common it is. On a daily basis, I spotted meals that were 'suitable for vegetarians' because they didn't contain meat or fish. What's more, the conversations were with non-veggies too.

"I always eat eggs and spinach for breakfast."
"Whenever I eat pizza at a restaurant, I always get vegetable because it tastes nicer."
"Sometimes I go all week without eating meat or fish and don't even realise."
"If I cook a curry at home, I never put meat or fish in because it lasts longer without it."
"When I'm on the go and have to grab a sandwich from the supermarket, I usually get cheese or egg. I never get one with meat or fish because it tastes nothing like either."

The strange thing was, these people would never proclaim they were eating a vegetarian meal, because they hadn't even realised. I started to wonder whether people who approached their nutritional choices this way would consider an all-out veggie diet someday. As I hadn't told anyone that I was in the veggie stage myself, I felt comfortable asking people, knowing they'd feel at ease and that I wasn't trying to convert them! When I asked, many of the responses to the veggie diet were along the same lines.

"But you need to have some meat in your diet."
"I don't really care about it that much."
"I'd be worried about eating more carbs."
"I'd hate to be that awkward person who moans at a restaurant if they didn't have anything on the menu."
"Sometimes I eat meat and fish to be easy, even though I'd rather not."

There were a lot of perceived barriers such as inconvenience, but many of these seemed to be brought about by 'overthinking' it. Similar to what I'd done when I went for breakfast at the cafe, so I wasn't one to judge.

Mostly, it seemed that people really didn't care about being associated with a "title" such as vegetarian. They just got on with it, eating veggie-friendly meals when they fancied it. Not having a title meant there was no pressure, and it seemed non-restrictive and more convenient.

"Vegetarian: ancient tribal name for the village idiot who can't hunt, fish, or light fires"

The first time I saw this was on Facebook. There was a meme that spread like wildfire through my feed as people commented, liked, and shared it. Without a doubt, there was an element of banter behind this misconception. But it's concerning that some people saw the meme and thought it was true!

The real history of vegetarianism is said to go back to ancient times (BC). The earliest records suggest that Egypt, India, and Greek civilisations in Italy and Greece had a diet closely connected to a non-violent attitude to animals. This was promoted by religious groups and philosophers.

Some of the earliest reliable evidence for vegetarian theory and practice in Greece dates from Pythagoras' lifetime, a philosopher and mathematician based in southern Italy. While he wished to avoid animal cruelty, he also saw the health benefits of a meat-free diet, so he abstained from it.

Pythagoras viewed vegetarianism as a key factor in peaceful human co-existence, putting forward the view that slaughtering animals brutalised the human soul. This tied into his beliefs on the subject of mysticism. In being a vegetarian, Pythagoras may have been trying to achieve a higher state of consciousness.

If you're not familiar with this, mysticism means any kind of ecstasy or altered state of consciousness that's given a religious or spiritual meaning. It also refers to attaining insight into ultimate or hidden truths, and to human transformation through various practices and experiences. This might be where the "hippy" label for veggies and vegans stems from.

Among other ideals that tied into mysticism, abstention from meat was a hallmark of the so-called "Pythagorean way of life" aka "Pythagoreanism", with followers known as "Pythagoreans". You could say this is the equivalent to "vegetarianism" and "vegetarians", or "veganism" and "vegans".

Going by the majority opinion in society, Pythagoreans were despised, perceived as troublemakers, and often had to keep their vegetarianism to themselves for fear of persecution. They apparently found very limited sympathy within the brutality of Ancient Rome, where many wild animals were killed at the hands of gladiators in the name of sport and spectacle.

In more recent history, vegetarianism was previously described as "the vegetable diet". It's thought that the name "vegetarian" came about in the mid-1800s in the UK, and was coined with the creation of the Vegetarian Society in Manchester in 1847. That pretty much disproves the misconception, as the 1800s doesn't seem like a very ancient tribal time, does it?

No flesh = peace of mind

It took a while to sink in that I'd been meat- and fish-free for the longest time in my entire life. Until this lightbulb moment, I hadn't truly acknowledged the reality that I wouldn't be eating dead animals anymore. I realised this while driving one day:

"I haven't eaten meat or fish for a while,
which means I haven't eaten an animal for a while,
which means I haven't tasted blood or flesh for a while,
which means nothing had to die to feed me for a while,
which must mean that I am saving animals every time
I don't eat them."

When I realised this was a logical explanation of the result of my actions, I felt a surge of euphoria. Up to then, I hadn't given myself credit on the magnitude of my actions—simply by swapping a few things in my diet, it could have such a wide effect elsewhere. I was so proud that I'd had a positive influence on something other than myself, and using only a fork! I thought:

"I choose to eat plant-based foods instead of animals...
I get healthier and animals don't have to die to feed me...
I win, and animals win. It's a WIN-WIN for
everyone/everything!"

Ultimately, I had peace of mind because of this logic. Even to this day, I feel as though I'm achieving something every time I eat, and that I'm contributing to others in the process. It was, and still is, a great vibe to have in day-to-day life, and that vibe feeds into other things. The best way to describe it is that it feels like progress, and progress is one of the things that makes me happy.

"Humans have evolved to eat meat and animal products"

The digestive system is very complex, and there are many examples that point towards how a human might not be best naturally suited to, or evolved to digest meats and animal products.

For example, a carnivore's stomach secretes powerful digestive enzymes, with up to 10 times the amount of hydrochloric acid than a human or herbivore has. This can kill many harmful microorganisms that may have been swallowed with the raw food killed or scavenged by the animal.

Bacteria such as E. coli, salmonella, campylobacter, and other pathogens would not survive in the stomach of a carnivore, whereas they can kill a human. This means that humans have to kill these bacteria outside the body through laborious cooking methods prior to eating the meat, while raw meat poses a significant risk.

This is just one example, but perhaps the most telling and significant proof that humans haven't yet evolved to eat meat and animal products, even if they have the technology and accessibility, is the fact that cholesterol contributes to atherosclerosis in humans.

Atherosclerosis occurs when fatty material called "atheroma" builds up in the lining of your artery walls and narrows your arteries. Your arteries are a system of tubes that transport blood around your body. Over time, the atheroma may grow bigger—until your arteries become so narrow that they can't let enough blood through. This can lead to angina, which is a sign that your heart isn't getting enough blood.

There are several causes of atherosclerosis including high cholesterol, which can clog up your arteries over time; high blood pressure, which can damage your artery walls over time; and, smoking, which can damage your arteries. If a fatty deposit breaks down or ruptures, a blood clot can form around it, which can also block your artery. This can lead to sudden death. If this artery supplies blood to the heart, it can cause a heart attack. If the artery supplies blood to the brain, this can cause a stroke.

Studies show that at least 2.6 million people in the UK have atherosclerosis and most people don't know they have it until they get symptoms such as angina, or have a heart attack or stroke. There is thought to be no known cure for atherosclerosis. That said, medical professionals are finding more ways to treat it. The recommendation is that the sooner you start these, the better.

One of the "treatments" is to reduce saturated fat in your diet, as this can raise 'bad' LDL cholesterol levels. This type of fat is found predominately in animal foods and products, such as all types of meat, eggs, and dairy.

Soluble fibre can slow the absorption of cholesterol and reduce the amount of cholesterol made by the liver. There is no fibre in any animal foods or products unless combined with plant-based foods. Oats, apples, and okra are sources of soluble fibre.

Other ways to prevent atherosclerosis worsening include avoiding smoking, exercising more, reducing stress levels, achieving a healthy weight, and turning to a fully plant-based diet.

This diet is well-known as being the best for lowering cholesterol, as no meat or animal products are consumed at all. Essentially, it is the only diet that includes no cholesterol and no animal fat. It won't necessarily reverse atherosclerosis, but it will prevent the build-up of fatty material from getting worse.

Atherosclerosis only affects herbivores, as it doesn't develop in omnivores and carnivores. The connection between cholesterol and atherosclerosis is strong. Cholesterol comes from animals and their products. Therefore, if we don't eat animals and their products, we don't take in cholesterol.

- Carnivore: metabolises large amounts of cholesterol.
- Omnivore: metabolises large amounts of cholesterol.
- Herbivore: metabolises small amounts of cholesterol.
- Human: metabolises small amounts of cholesterol.

I was a BAD (unhealthy) veggie

Eww, it pains to me to say this... but it's so true. All personal standards towards my health went haywire. Perhaps the worst since my travelling days a few years back. Maybe because it was midway in the journey, or because I didn't know any better (I did). Either way, I sincerely hope that anyone who attempts a plant-based diet does the veggie stage more healthily than I did! It helps to be aware of the potential flaws that can happen at this stage.

When I technically became a "vegetarian", my mindset changed. I began to think differently, and my diet went skew-whiff. All the foundations I had set before the journey began to change for the worse. I felt unhealthier than ever. For some reason, I felt like being a veggie was an invitation to eat any food, so long as it was classed as "veggie-friendly". In my mind, this gave me the green light to crack on regardless of whether it was healthy or not.

Instead of plant-based options that are suitable for veggies, I was proactively eating more processed food than ever before. I was most partial to bread, cheese, whey protein flapjacks, and chocolate. I still believed (or was lying to myself) that eggs and cheese were better sources of protein than plant-based foods. This meant I ate more animal products—regardless of my gut feeling to eat less of them due to their high saturated fat content.

A few weeks into the veggie stage, the proven foundation of a wide variety of nutritious fruit and veg had been replaced with stodge. I was barely eating any of the good stuff and wasn't even having smoothies anymore. After a while, my body began to change, but in my head I was like: "It's okay."

Then, I read a survey from the U.S. that half of people aged

50 years and older wished they had more strength or energy to participate in the activities they enjoy. I really didn't want to reach that stage! Call me crazy, but I'd gone from feeling so energised in all walks of life to suddenly needing to reassure myself that I wasn't losing everything I'd worked so hard for. I wasn't exercising much due to writing the book, and I knew that if I kept eating so much junk food, it would show quicker than if I was working out. Not just in a superficial way either, but in my overall aura.

I was being naive, knowing I needed to turn it around asap, but losing confidence in my ability to make it to a plant-based diet. I also knew that to turn it around, all I had to do was lock down the foundation I'd had for years: food prep, and build on my diet from there. But for some reason, I just felt like I couldn't do it. Instead, I was happy opting for a quick fix to "get by". This vicious cycle continued for some time before I could snap myself out of it.

"Most vegetarians are unhealthy"

In the mainstream, there is conflicting evidence on whether the veggie diet is healthy or unhealthy. One 2014 study was so point-blank against the vegetarian diet that people raised qualms about it being suspicious. The publication had to justify that it wasn't released just to promote the meat industry.

Before believing what you read about overall diets, I reiterate that whether a diet is healthy or unhealthy depends on the individual's nutritional decisions over an extended period of time. It's not the diet—it's the individual.

When it comes to studies, are they reporting on health-conscience people who don't eat meat—or someone who fills up on milk, cheese, eggs, then eats a few fruit and vegetables? If the latter, then proclaiming to the world that vegetarians are unhealthy because meat isn't in their diet is absurd.

Like any diet, a veggie diet can be unhealthy if you're not eating the right foods. However, even experienced coaches who deal with nutrition in the mainstream are stuck when it comes to promoting a healthy veggie diet. I know a PT who did a diet plan for a vegetarian client once and literally replaced meat with Quorn for every meal. When I asked why, they said "because Quorn is the only lean protein that I knew of that isn't meat or fish." I'm not saying Quorn is unhealthy, but where's the variety of nutritious, plant-based foods that can also account for protein intake? As well as lack of knowledge, a veggie diet can be unhealthy due to:

- A tendency to snack on veggie-friendly junk foods.
- A reliance on the same foods day in day out.
- A desire to not eat plant-based foods.
- A tendency to overeat animal products.

To have a healthy veggie diet, the glycemic index (aka GI) is useful. It can help build your confidence as you transition from this stage. It's what I used to reign myself in when I was at my most unhealthy. It generally gets you eating more single-ingredient foods and fibre to keep you fuller for longer.

The concept of GI was apparently developed back in the 80s and had it's heyday in the mainstream. However, when I first got into the health and fitness industry in 2007, it was still being mentioned. For the past few years, talk of GI in the mainstream has been relatively quiet.

GI is the glycemic index of food, and it's measured on a scale of 0-100 (lowest to highest) representing the total rise in a person's blood sugar level following the consumption of food. Basically, the higher the GI, the higher your blood sugar levels post-consumption, and vice versa for a low GI. This means that high-GI types of food are metabolised more quickly and so tend to make you feel hungry again sooner.

Foods with a low GI are popularly known as "slow release" energy, and foods with a high GI are known as "fast release" energy. Following these principles, people tend to consume slow release carbs around sedentary times in their day and fast release carbs around activity. Here are some examples:

Low G.I = foods with a GI range of 55 or less

- Beans: Most beans, including black, pinto, kidney, lentils, and chickpeas.
- Seeds: Sunflower, flax, pumpkin, poppy, sesame, and hemp.
- Nuts: Most nuts, including walnuts, cashews, and peanuts.
- Grains: Most intact grains, including oat, rye, rice, barley, millet, durum wheat, spelt wheat, and kamut (Khorasan or oriental) wheat.
- Vegetables: Most vegetables.
- Fruits: Most fruits, peaches, strawberries, and mangoes.

Medium G.I = foods with a GI range of 56-69

- Pitta bread, basmati rice, brown rice, grape juice, raisins, prunes, dried apricots, cranberry juice, orange juice, wholemeal bread, and bananas.

High G.I = foods with a GI range of 70 and above

- Dextrose, grape sugar, high fructose corn syrup, white bread, white rice, commercial cereals, maltodextrin, potatoes, white bagels, and cakes.

Veggie vs. Pescy

Although dropping fish seemed like the natural thing to do at the time, I struggled to keep up my motivation when fish dropped out completely. When this kind of thing happens, you can begin to get cynical of "the diet" you're currently doing, rather than your own diet. When times got hard and unhealthy, I debated whether being "a vegetarian who eats fish" is better than being "a vegetarian who doesn't eat fish"!

Then I realised. As a pescatarian, I had to cook the fish and garnish it. I'd always believed that because the fish was "fresh", the most suitable garnish was fresh vegetables and salad. It was clear that the "freshness" had gone from my diet—and freshness would get me back on track. I was hoping to apply my fresh theory to plant-based foods: "fresh attracts fresh".

It was time to start buying fresh food, cooking it from scratch, prepping it, trying new recipes, and going in a different direction. No more blaming "the veggie diet" for my diet!

The first thing I did was cook large "bang for your buck" type meals such as vegetable curries and stews. I picked these types of meals because they required little effort to prepare and would last for a few days. There was very little hassle in making these meals, so I hoped that having something accessible and already prepared would far outweigh the temptation of eating convenient, stodgy foods, because they would be just as convenient.

I began to include lentils in curries and quinoa in stews. This accounted for my protein intake rather than cheese and eggs. These plant-based foods were saving my body of a lot of saturated fat in place of the old guard! It was hard to get my head around having a plant-based protein that contained carbs as a main source of protein, but when I started to feel the benefits of eating fresh food again, I didn't give it much more thought.

It was the first time I had gone about cooking without the "protein" to go with it, and what I mean is animal protein, because my old self had seen it that way. I used to believe that you had to include animal protein in a meal to get the best from it, regardless of the plant-based protein included.

After a few meals like this, the "natural" feeling had come back to me and I felt that I was on the right road to a plant-based diet again. It was obvious that the "eat anything because its veggie-friendly" mindset wasn't the way to go, because I'd felt like shit! I can understand why so many people who try a veggie diet go back to meat or fish, because they're put their faith in "the vegetarian diet" and not their own diet.

"People have lived to be over 100 and they eat meat and animal products, so it's all down to luck"

In recent mainstream news, and coincidently around the time that the World Health Organisation (WHO) shed light on red and processed meat being harmful to health, there was a story of a lady in the U.S. who is one of only two living people born in the 1800s. Aged 116 (at the time of writing this), she puts her long life down to eating bacon and eggs every morning for over a century. A sign on her kitchen wall apparently reads "Bacon makes everything better!" She also cited not smoking or drinking, and getting "lots of sleep" as other reasons for her longevity. She had no children, but her niece said she grew up in a rural town eating fruit and vegetables that she picked herself, as fresh and organic as could be.

This isn't just an isolated, exceptional case where someone consumed animal products daily and lived to be over 100. The oldest living person in Europe attributed her longevity to eating several raw eggs every day. These people are of course amazing in reaching these milestones; however, some animal eaters focus on these cases and neglect the other statistics and factors that actually go against longevity and eating animal products.

Although there is no dead-set way to live to be 100, there are a few consistencies that play into potentially living longer. Unsurprisingly, these are things that most people consider to be common sense if you want to be healthier.

For example, it was recently found that common bad habits such as smoking, drinking too much alcohol, not exercising, and not eating much fruit and veg can reduce your life expectancy by as many as 12 years. Other lifestyle habits such as a positive outlook appear consistently in many people who live long lives. However, it's also no guarantee, and I'm sure we all know someone who had a positive outlook but sadly passed away regardless.

So, is living longer really down to the luck of the draw? Should you eat meat and animal products because you enjoy them, and because you're going to die at some point anyway?

- According to a 2016 report, the average life expectancy in the UK is 81 years. Monaco has the highest, at a reported 90 years for men and women combined. Japan is third, with 85 years combined. The U.S. comes in at 42nd with 80 years, and the UK is 30th of 224 countries.

- There's an estimated 316,600 centenarians worldwide, and women tend to live longer than men. A study found that for every 100 women aged 60, there were 84 men. For every 100 women aged 80 or over, there are 61 men. The proportion of women to men continues to rise with age.

- Coronary heart disease (CHD) is the leading cause of death in the UK and worldwide. It's responsible for more than 73,000 deaths in the UK each year. Around 1 in 6 men and 1 in 10 women die from CHD.

- The difference between men and women could be due to gender differences in psychosocial and behavioural coronary risk factors, including excessive alcohol consumption and smoking, favouring women. Overall, it appears that men's ability to cope with stressful events may be less adaptive physiologically, behaviourally, and emotionally, contributing to their increased risk of CHD.

Statistically, a vegan or vegetarian diet can help people live longer. A collection of data found that a vegetarian and vegan diet could even contribute to around an extra lifespan of 4-10 years more than a meat eater!

The NHS atlas of risk can help to put health risks and death rates into perspective in the UK. From the highest contributor of death risk to the lowest in order, they are:

1. Heart and circulatory disorders.
2. Cancer.
3. Respiratory disorders.
4. Digestive disorders.
5. Kidney infections.
6. Infections.
7. Non-transport accidents.
8. Diabetes.
9. Musculoskeletal disorders.
10. Suicide.
11. Transport accidents.
12. Mental health disorders.
13. Undetermined events.
14. Murder.
15. Medical complications.
16. Pregnancy and birth.
17. War.

Undoubtedly, an accident or an onset of a previous lifestyle choice (such as smoking) could strike at any time. However, going by these findings, it appears that you can reduce your risk of diseases that may cause an earlier death. Going through this list, I linked diet alone to around 10 of these causes of death—in particular the higher rankings.

Outside of uncontrollable circumstances such as accidents, you can increase your chances of living longer by adhering to "man-made" controllable factors such as eating healthily, getting regular exercise, and avoiding bad habits such as smoking and alcohol.

Processes in poultry and dairy

Before getting involved in it myself, my opinion on the veggie diet was that people were only veggies because they cared about animals and didn't want to put another living, sentient being through any suffering. When I adopted the diet myself and spoke to others about it, this did turn out to be true in many cases. However, some people just didn't like the taste or texture of meat, and didn't think about the ethical side of it that much.

When I looked into veggie food more specifically, the information I found was a lot deeper and more sinister than I'd bargained for. I'd assumed that "vegetarian-friendly" sources of food meant no physical or mental harm to the animal. However, when I looked into the dairy and poultry processes, the animals seemed to be put through equal—if not more—suffering than being killed for meat. Morally, it was as bad as it gets. Then I realised that the dairy industry is the meat industry, because every cow that produces milk becomes meat eventually. And the poultry industry is the meat industry, because every chicken that lays eggs becomes meat eventually too.

As this stage was so current to me, all the research and information really hit home. I saw very early on that the vegetarians who don't eat meat because they care about animals may not have researched what the dairy and poultry processes entail. If they did, they may want to go plant-based asap. I realised that even for some vegetarians, there is a lack of association between the process and the product. As the old saying goes, "ignorance is bliss."

When looking at meat or fish on a plate, some people tend not to think about how it got there. If that's the case for a blatant piece of flesh in a see-through packet, just imagine how far removed your brain, and ultimately your morals, get from a chocolate bar, cheese, or a protein flapjack. Unless you take the time to look into how this gets there, you just wouldn't know. The marketing and packaging of products these days is very clever. Things can seem way more fun than what they actually are! One thing is for sure, after I acknowledged the association between the process and the product, I was ready to move forward. And I wasn't deterred by what people think of a plant-based diet—I was moving to the next stage.

"Free range eggs and organic dairy is humane"

Although slightly more humane, "free range" or "organic" doesn't quite mean these processes are "humane". Whichever way you look at it, the animal involved is being extorted for some sort of gain—and let's face it, not their own. Come the end of their tenure, when they can't provide any more gain for others, the end result ultimately climaxes in their death, and they're turned into meat for someone to feed on. Whichever way they are killed, they are killed. Simple as that.

The definition of "free range" is: Of livestock, especially poultry, kept in natural conditions, with freedom of movement.

Chickens on free-range farms often endure the same mutilations as those on conventional factory farms. This can include debeaking without painkillers. You can probably imagine this doesn't feel very nice for them. Male chicks are usually killed at birth, as they don't produce eggs and are therefore deemed useless. The slightly more humane aspect vs. caging procedures is that they might have access to outdoor areas. However, it isn't specified how much time they spend outside or how much space they should be given to be considered "free range". Most of the time, they are shacked up with many other chickens, confined to a crowded shed, and possibly covered in faeces.

The definition of "organic" is: Of food or farming methods, produced or involving production without the use of chemical fertilisers, pesticides, or other artificial chemicals.

It has been reported that cows on organic dairy farms may also be kept in crowded sheds, also coated in faeces. The process of how the milk, and therefore dairy products, come about is the same. They are artificially impregnated by a human, and their calves are taken from them soon after birth, sometimes right in front of their eyes. I'm no cow scientist, but this must cause intense emotional stress to the mother and baby. Think of it this way, an animal has to give birth to produce milk.

Cows on organic farms often aren't given antibiotics, even when they're sick or when their udders become infected, which happens often. They can't be treated because medicated animals lose their "organic" status. Even if they were given antibiotics, would you want to put that in your body—second-hand cow medicine?

Economically, these so-called "more humane practices" are usually more expensive! So the less harm the animal has to endure, the more expensive? Bizarre, the true cost of compassion!

Here, I'm talking more about mainstream farms. I understand that some farms may go about their practices differently, and should you decide to look into this yourself, you will see. Overall though, the same things pretty much go down. The animal will be extorted until it is no longer efficient and is then killed for another use.

When you've done some further research into it and made up your own mind, you might choose to boycott the whole thing and keep the boundaries of health, ethics, and your economical budget unscathed and unblurred. That way, there are no compromises. And, you won't need to wonder about what is more humane.

Christmas without the turkey

Christmas: the one time of year in the UK when it's pretty much mandatory to go out and buy a turkey to eat on Christmas day. It was going to be a rebellious day for someone with a vegetarian appetite, and who has aspirations for a plant-based diet in the near future! Given that I wouldn't be cooking the dinner, I had to tread carefully in making my preferences known. I needed to come across as grateful, but also have my intentions known. My nan would doing the cooking for my family, so it was her I had to confide in!

I said to her in a loving way: "Naaaaaaaaan, thank you so much for putting all of this together for everyone today. I'm really appreciative, and you know I love your cooking more than anyone's. I hope you won't be offended, but I'm not going to have any meat with my dinner today because I've recently gone onto a vegetarian diet and I'm feeling really good about it. I hope you don't mind?"

She replied in a very open manner: "Vegetarian! You?" Not to worry darling, I won't be offended. More for everyone else!" She then said in a disappointed manner: "What are you going to have instead though? I would have done it for you!"

I replied: "I'm just going to literally take the turkey out and maybe eat more veg instead—I don't want to make a big fuss. That's if there's enough left over that is. If not, no worries. I'll survive!"

She agreed there would be and that was it. Problem solved. I had faced my biggest challenge on my journey so far and had massively broken tradition. But I found a solution that made me and my nan happy. Things were a little different at the dinner table mind you, as I got some banter from the rest of my family about why there was no turkey on my plate.

I smiled and laughed my way through it, giving whatever I could back to them! I told them I was trying something new for work, as a bit of an "experiment", which felt quite fitting because it kind of was. And it gave me peace of mind because I wasn't lying to them. I also managed to keep the details out, so I didn't come across as preachy.

Judging by everyone's reactions, they were more intrigued than critical about the whole thing. It seemed that by staying quietly confident in my knowledge and keeping my cards close to my chest about my aim, this helped my family to "get it".

Despite my apprehensions about Christmas dinner without the turkey, the meal was still incredible! And it was the only Christmas dinner that I didn't feel that bloated, hot, and full-up after feeling from the copious amounts of meat. Plant-based foods thankfully don't have that "meat sweats" effect.

However, that non-bloated feeling was ruined when it came to dessert. I had my old favourite, Christmas pudding with brandy butter. The butter contained dairy, which was fine with the vegetarian title. Still, I considered not eating it, but I really bloody wanted it at the time.

Nobody questioned the fact that I was eating dairy, and I didn't have to explain it to everyone. In fact, my family seemed quite happy that I was getting involved, and it made the veggie thing more "normal" to them.

"Christmas isn't Christmas without the turkey. Just like Easter isn't Easter without the Easter eggs"

When it comes to seasonal events such as Christmas or Easter, many people are sentimental about the traditions of these events. Even if you're not sentimental about them, you've probably enjoyed turkey at Christmas and a chocolate Easter egg at Easter before.

The funny thing is, although we engage in these events, not everyone actually likes them. A reported 1 in 5 people in the UK don't like Christmas, and 1 in 6 wish they could cancel it! Despite this, the majority of people still partake in some of the traditional elements such as having turkey for dinner.

The same can be said of Easter. Apparently, 53% of children don't even know the meaning of Easter or why it exists. But the majority of kids wouldn't say no to an Easter egg. Their parents might not know the meaning either, but encourage the tradition of purchasing chocolate eggs for their kids.

In 2016, 15 million turkeys were killed and of those, 10 million were just for Christmas (according to Bernard Matthews), meaning the rest of the year, it's barely being consumed in comparison.

76% of UK households will be eating it on the day (and maybe lunch the next day). But how many of these people only do this because of tradition?

Likewise, over Easter weekend, it's tradition that eggs "must" be eaten. Over just one weekend out of 52 in the year, Easter eggs reportedly make up 10% of the UK's annual spending on chocolate. Around 80 million Easter eggs are sold annually in the UK alone, an average of two per person. People just love them, but only on that weekend!

These statistics show that people seem to enjoy and choose these foods, but more so on these particular dates. And we know that sentiment, habit, and tradition play a big role in how much these dates mean to people. People look forward to all the traditional elements that come with these occasions. However, it's just as easy to replace these "traditional foods" with something else. For example, that Christmas, I had a dairy-free advent calendar.

Should you decide not to abide by these traditions, there is undoubtedly an element of change required. There is a national fixation on these dates as if they are "do or die", as if you're a "weirdo" if you don't do what everyone else is doing. However, you're going to be a "weirdo" every day in not abiding by the tradition of consuming animals and animal products on a daily basis, so what difference does Christmas and Easter make? It's up to you to decide what standard you wish to hold your own diet by.

Tree hugger potential?

As New Year's Eve drew to a close, rather than doing what I had always done and reflecting on the year gone by, I started to look ahead...

I had procrastinated a bit about moving to the next stage—mostly vegan—but after writing my goals for the year, I was more excited and confident to move on to the next stage of the journey than ever before! I was genuinely excited about the potential benefits and knock-on effects on my life and others. Moving on to a mostly vegan diet would bring a host of new restrictions and inconveniences that I would have to adapt to, and also a different identity in society. Very almost the "V word"!

Due to the sheer reality that some people associated "vegan" with a certain type of person, I knew I had to tread carefully in taking the next steps forward, more so than ever. I didn't resent people for this prejudice because they genuinely didn't know any better about the subject. But I didn't want to encounter any extreme changes in my social life or my career at this stage.

I've never hated on vegans, but until I started looking into a plant-based diet and saw how "normal" and natural it was, my general impression was your typical mainstream idea of a vegan: a scruffy, poor, eco-warrior, protester, outlaw, weed/roll-up smoker, semi-alcoholic, awkward pain in the backside kind of div. Basically the opposite of what is considered "cool", "normal", or even "acceptable" by mainstream society. It was considered weird to many.

It's hard to say exactly how many vegans there are, as I've never been asked the question for a study, so I imagine there are many others such as myself who are unaccounted for. But because of these statistics, you can expect people to become, well, inquisitive about the vegan thing.

Back when I first stopped eating meat, someone said to me: "You're not going to become one of those 'vegans' are you?" Thanks to the aptly titled 'Mostly Vegan' stage, which is still technically vegetarian, I was able to not come across as so vegan until I'd made a few changes to my diet and felt confident enough to live with it openly in society. You'll find that sometimes, you have to adjust the way you do things because of how it's seen in the eyes of others. It's not that you should let someone's ideology of something control your life though—it's just so you can patiently build your understanding of how to go about your diet first.

"All vegans are the same – bloody hippies!"

The first "vegan" I ever saw was on Coronation Street. Don't judge me... it makes me laugh that I remember this so well, because I never really knew why. Back in the day, I used to stay at my grandparents a lot. My nan was a big fan of the soap and she used to watch it like clockwork. I was around 9 years old and was most likely playing on my Game Boy in the same room as her while it was on, so not even fully watching it.

They introduced a character called "Spider", who was your classic mainstream impression of a vegan. What struck me as significant about this character, and took my eyes off my Game Boy for a second, was that he was asking the weirdest questions. Questions that at the time I had no idea could even be asked, let alone answered. For some reason, the question that really got my attention was when someone offered him a glass of water, and he asked whether it was "hard or soft water".

I looked at my nan and was like, "Naaaaaaan, what's the difference between hard and soft water?" And she said, "I have no idea."

From that moment on, every time this "Spider" character was in a scene, I took notice because I was intrigued and found him unpredictable. Not once did it cross my mind that in a bizarre twist of fate, I would be looking into a vegan diet one day. Quite the opposite actually, because he wasn't exactly selling it to me! My only insight into a vegan lifestyle at this point was "Spider's lifestyle", which put me off anything vegan for a long time! It was too weird and "out there" for me to even comprehend at the tender age of 9.

It's apparent that due to the lack (or rightful portrayal of) of vegans in mainstream society, the rare ones you come across will absolutely have an impact on you and fine-tune your way of thinking in the future. This is something to think about if you make it to the final stage of the diet yourself.

Say from experience that like me, you've been left believing that all vegans are hippies. Ask yourself, are they? The answer = no. Clearly not. Over the years, I have met more self-proclaimed hippies who eat meat and animal products than those who don't.

Trying to say that all vegans are the same, and categorising them in society by their perceived preference, is like trying to say that all animal eaters are the same and have the same interests too... "Those animal eaters. They're all bloody non-hippies!" It just doesn't work, does it?!

VEGETARIAN summary

The vegetarian/vegan label doesn't guarantee it's healthy.

Although accessible and highlighted at times, make nutritional decisions based on suitability for this stage and nutritional content—not just suitability.

Keep an eye out for other vegetarians in society.

The likelihood of meeting another veggie is quite likely these days. Realise that some people are mostly veggie without even noticing it themselves. Take note of when people are eating vegetarian-friendly meals without even mentioning it.

Make carbs work for you by timing them around activity levels.

If your reason for not wanting to eat plant-based proteins that contain carbs is because you're worried about carbs, you can account for this by either: increasing activity (output) or consuming less carbohydrates elsewhere in your day-to-day diet (input).

Break the seal.

If at any point you fall off the wagon and begin to create unhealthy habits, kickstart new, healthier ones as soon as you get the inclination that you could do better. The longer you leave it, the harder it is to get back on track.

Fresh attracts fresh.

The more fresh food you decide to prepare and eat, the more likely you will keep this up. And dare I say it, the more you'll enjoy the process more because you feel better. This works the other way too—junk food/poor nutritional decisions make you feel like shit. Choose wisely.

Carbs attract carbs.

If you think that carbs are evil, it might be because they make you want to eat more of them. Create a demand for energy through exercise and daily activity levels to feel a greater peace of mind when consuming them. Then you'll feel like you've earned them.

For some, ignorance is bliss.

Many people have no idea where their food comes from in any detail, yet they're happy to keep going the way they are. Without doing further research, they take it for face value and hope that it is what they hope it is. You needn't be the one to tell them it isn't.

Treat seasonal meals like any other meals.

No meal has to be on a pedestal, where it's mandatory that you have to eat it that way or eat it at all. When it comes to things like Christmas dinner, make it work for you, even if it means being a bit different to everyone else.

Don't eat the non-vegan-friendly ingredient.

If you're at a meal and you don't fancy eating meat or any other animal products, then don't. If you haven't got a suitable replacement with you, just eat more of what you can as a replacement.

Some people find the "V word" offensive.

Come to terms with the fact that some people have their mind made up that vegan stuff is stupid. Regardless of whether they have ever looked into it or met one face to face! Try to avoid mentioning this word until you are confident in your diet and talking about it.

Stage Four
MOSTLY VEGAN

No more chocolate unless it's vegan friendly! And trying pizza without the cheese—WTF!

Over Christmas, I'd consumed my fair share of chocolate and was pretty sick of it! So I figured the first simple swap of this stage should be here. It was quite lucky, because Christmas was one of the rare times I eat chocolate as a treat, usually avoiding it for health reasons. Plus, most people are looking for a health kick in the New Year anyway.

You may have a sweeter tooth than I do, so this may be a harder swap for you. However, vegan-friendly chocolate isn't that difficult to come by these days, even in mainstream supermarkets. You'll be surprised by just how many chocolate products are suitable for vegans or are 100% plant-based. These products often have coconut or soy milk in place of cow's milk, so they may be marketed as something else in the mainstream, such as "dairy-free".

The "V word" can be a turn-off for prospective customers, so some companies avoid the subject on their packaging. For example, there are "accidental" vegan-friendly chocolate products, where a company hasn't used any animal products in the recipe, but hasn't mentioned it either. The same goes for other foods and sweets. You can find a list of these on many different websites if you type 'accidental vegan food' into Google. Theres also a page dedicated to it on Instagram **@accidentlyveganuk**.

Classically, most vegan-friendly chocolate that you come across in the mainstream is likely to be a dark variety. Dark chocolate tends to have a higher content of cacao as the main ingredient, and doesn't always use milk in the recipe. Dark chocolate has become another addition to many 'superfood' lists in recent years, as cacao is known to provide antioxidants.

The same can't be said of other chocolate varieties, such as brown (aka milk) and white chocolate, as they tend not to be so transparent about their cacao content and glorify "milkier" and "smoother" in the description. These factors are often a dead giveaway in whether something is vegan-friendly or not.

So, switching chocolate wasn't so difficult for me. Then came pizza. Pizza is one of my favourite foods of all time and I had it at least once a week. It was a dream to behold post training. I would really work hard during my workout if I knew that pizza was my reward. The thing is though, pizza = cheese. Cheese = dairy. And its association to the processes of dairy was a bit more obvious than the shiny packaging of chocolate.

One night, I'd decided on pizza for dinner. I'd never made my own at this stage, so I ordered a takeaway. I ordered a large vegetable pizza from Domino's without the cheese. I genuinely believed it would be a massive pain in the arse to get hold of one, but it was extremely easy!

The pizza arrived and it looked and smelt just like any "normal" pizza that has cheese. It also tasted better in my opinion, because it wasn't greasy, and it didn't bloat me out. I knew I'd eaten a pizza after it, but I didn't have that "I've just stuffed my face and now I'm in a carb coma" feeling that you get after some takeaways.

I used to think it was the cheese that made a pizza. But for me, I've realised it's actually the topping, the base, and the sauce... everything but the cheese! The same could be said for chocolate— I used to think it was the milk that made it. But it turned out to be the cacao and all the other ingredients.

"I couldn't give up animal products because I love chocolate too much"

When it comes to actual cravings for chocolate, 40% of women in the U.S. report having chocolate cravings, compared to just 15% of men. In fact, half of the women in this report craved chocolate specifically around menstruation. Companies capitalise on this by marketing chocolate as a way for women to deal with negative emotions such as mood swings and depression that may come with PMS (premenstrual syndrome).

Eating chocolate is thought to increase the level of endorphins released in the brain, giving strength to the claim that chocolate is a "comfort food". These endorphins work to lessen pain and decrease stress. When we consume chocolate, our brain releases a neurotransmitter called serotonin, which is known to be an anti-depressant. So, there is a reason why chocolate relieves PMS.

One of the chemicals that causes the release of serotonin is an amino acid called tryptophan. Besides chocolate, it's also found in animals and animal products, which may explain our dependency on these foods. However, there are also plant-based sources of tryptophan such as: tofu, spirulina, soy beans, wheatgerm, oat bran, and seeds including pumpkin, sunflower, chia, sesame, and hemp.

One of the more unique neurotransmitters released by chocolate is phenylethylamine. It's known to improve mood and decrease depression. In fact, it's even called the "love drug" in the mainstream because it makes your pulse rate increase, resulting in a similar feeling to being in love! Hence: "I couldn't give up animal products because I love chocolate too much."

In the UK alone, an estimated 660,900 tonnes of chocolate are consumed each year, which is an average of 11kg per person annually, or around 3 bars each per week. Around half of the chocolate eaten in the world is consumed in Europe, and studies show that in countries with warmer climates, less chocolate is consumed. The UK, Switzerland, Germany, France, and Belgium (known to be the home of quality chocolate) ate considerably more than the sunnier Italy and Spain.

Around 66% of chocolate is consumed between meals (as snacks) and 22% between 8pm and midnight. Besides the link to PMS in women, these timings suggest chocolate is used to help people unwind and relax, such as the end of the day being a big one. If you know that your main chocolate consumption happens during these times, you can be prepared for it when you get the urge! Not that you have to give up chocolate completely, but you can get a vegan-friendly alternative ready for when the time comes.

Quite often, mainstream cocoa powder and chocolate have been chemically processed and roasted, which destroys a large amount of the antioxidants and flavonoids found in cacao, between 60-90%. Both are thought to reduce dangerous inflammation in the arteries and may lower blood pressure and cholesterol. Research shows that a diet rich in flavonoids is beneficial and its promotion is justifiable, although its full potential is not yet known. Dietary sources of flavonoids include fruits, vegetables, nuts, seeds, and spices.

A higher cacao content is usually found in dark chocolate, and it appears that many people are moving towards this more "healthy" option, marking the biggest growth area in the chocolate industry. Rest assured, you won't be considered a weirdo for going down this road! To get ahead of the curve, you can choose vegan-friendly too. To get all the benefits mentioned, look out for the cacao content and not those mainstream advertising gimmicks that play on your mood or seasonal trends. Other benefits of cacao include:

High in antioxidants

Exposure to the sun, cigarette smoke, pollution, and toxic chemicals (such as chemical weed killers and unhealthy foods) can all release free radical activity in the body. They are also produced by factors such as stress, and damage healthy tissue. Antioxidants in the foods you eat reverse this process, helping to combat disease and fight harmful free radicals.

Notable plant-based source of iron

One dark chocolate bar of 70%-85% cacao content (per 100g) = 11.9mg iron. X4 more than steak (2.9mg). X7 more than lamb chops (1.6mg) X4 more than spinach (2.7mg). Don't forget that vitamin C is said to increase absorption of iron.

Notable plant-based source of magnesium

We are told to take increased amounts of calcium in our diet as a supplement to prevent osteoporosis; however, without magnesium, calcium may not be fully utilised, and under-absorption problems may occur, leading to arthritis, osteoporosis, menstrual cramps, and some premenstrual symptoms.

Other plant-based examples of magnesium include: Rice bran, seaweed, basil, hemp seed, basil, coriander, chives, cumin, parsley, wheat bran, pumpkin seeds, blackstrap molasses, dill weed, flaxseed, chia seeds, brazil nuts and sesame seeds.

Experimenting with beans, pulses, and grains

Being English, I'd eaten Heinz Baked Beans many a time with fry ups, but I hadn't prepared many other styles of beans before this point. My consumption of pulses was even rarer. To be honest, my knowledge on beans and pulses was so dire that I genuinely thought a Heinz Baked Bean came from a bean known as the "Baked Bean". It wasn't until I looked into this that I realised they're actually made from haricot beans aka navy beans!

Although I'd always enjoyed eating various types of beans in a meal, in the past I'd put up boundaries against cooking them as I believed that beans:

- Were awkward to cook: Turns out they're ridiculously easy to cook and can be done so in abundance. Ideal for food prep!
- Make you fart: You'll read more on this in the next section.
- Contained carbs: This is true, however that's not a reason to not eat them considering their other health benefits.

I went online and looked into the different types of beans and pulses available, the benefits of each, why they would suit me, and how to bloody cook them! Then I started adding them to brown rice, stir fries, salads, and curries.

Adding beans and pulses was an extremely practical option for food prep and increased my protein intake—without having to add any animal products. My original choices were black beans, broad beans, edamame beans, lentils, and chickpeas. These days, I try to eat as many types as possible.

Then I did the same with grains. The two seemed to go hand in hand, nutritionally-speaking. They were both excellent sources of plant-based protein, high in fibre, and contained carbs that would provide slow-release energy.

There were a few grains that I'd always wished to use more of, but never did, for the same reasons as with beans. These were quinoa, wheatgerm, and barley. Annoyingly, I seemed to fall back on the most convenient, popular grains in the Western diet: wheat, oats, and rice. Especially wheat, as it was in pasta, cereals, and its most popular by-product (and my personal favourite) bread. I say "annoyingly", because it meant I was often eating more processed versions of grains.

My biggest concern when starting to include more grains in my diet, especially while not exercising so much, was the carb issue. I tended to store more fat when on a higher carb diet, especially when eating more processed than wholegrain carbs. Without getting too technical, the more exercise I did, the more carbs I could eat after exercise without going into a carb coma!

It wasn't until I reached the final stage—where I dropped the "carbs make you fat" concern and started to relax about it—that I started to fully enjoy grains for what they are. I began eating a variety of types instead of relying on wheat-based products for convenience. Reducing my portion sizes dependant on my daily activity also helped, focusing on my overall calories with all food in mind for the day. This gave me peace of mind as I adjusted.

"Beans, beans, they're good for your heart. The more you eat, the more you..."

You could easily assume that the famous farting side effects of beans may be due to their extremely high fibre content. The fibre also accounts for "the good for your heart" bit of the song. Fibre helps to improve blood cholesterol levels and lower the risk of heart disease, stroke, obesity, and type 2 diabetes. It would be a shame to avoid these potential benefits just because of the concern over farting! But is it the fibre alone that causes flatulence?

First of all, it's important to acknowledge why farting more is a cause of concern for some people. It can be seen as rude and disgusting to some people. These values can be made worse by the timing, volume, and smell of the fart, and can make people feel very uncomfortable! So, this might put some people off moving towards a plant-based diet.

At the dinner table, on public transport, or just before sex are probably known as the worst times to let a loud one go! Though I don't think there's ever an ideal time to let a smelly one go. Unless, it's away from people and out in the open, with a fast wind to take it away—as far as possible!

Some people find it more offensive than others, and this is completely dependent on the individual's perspective. Some people find them funny! It's worth noting that holding on to a fart can be just as uncomfortable, but in a different way. Holding them in can cause gas, bloating, pain, and other uncomfortable symptoms that can affect confidence and mobility.

Society paints farting as more of a "blokey" thing to do, and women are "supposed" to be a little more prudish on the subject. Contrary to what most people believe though, men and women are said to fart equally as much, with the average person farting 14 times a day. If you think this is way more than you do, most farts take place at night while you're sleeping, which you probably won't even know you're doing. Your partner might though.

Let's have a quick biology lesson. When your body digests food, it goes from the mouth to the oesophagus, then to the stomach, then the small intestine. The main function of the small intestine is to absorb nutrients and minerals from food. Following absorption, nutrients travel through the bloodstream to organs and tissues.

The food parts that are not absorbed go through the colon (large intestine), where they are later eliminated. In the small intestine, digestive enzymes break apart the bonds that connect various building blocks of foods. For example, pancreatic amylase breaks up oligosaccharides made from glucose into their glucose sub-units. However, certain oligosaccharides are built from other small sugars, and pancreatic amylase doesn't work on these. Two important examples are galacto-oligosaccharides and fructans:

- Galacto-oligosaccharides: Made of galactose, these sub-units are present in large quantities of beans, lentils, and chickpeas.
- Fructans: These strands of fructose sub-units are found in grains, especially wheat, rye, and barley, and veg such as onions, artichokes, and leeks.

It's thought that self-diagnosis of a gluten allergy, which leads to abstaining from all foods containing gluten, is often misconstrued based on an individual's ability to handle the breakdown process of these two (among others). Most people can handle modest amounts of grains and beans fairly well, some people can tolerate large amounts, and some people can't handle even a little bit. And any given person may handle galacto-oligosaccharides and fructans completely differently.

In either case, any undigested oligosaccharides pass through the small intestine into the colon and are eliminated from the body in poo. Upon reaching the colon, they will cause discomfort, such as bloating and diarrhoea.

With all that in mind, beans will make you fart more. That is true. But the amount that you can handle is purely dependant on your digestive capabilities. My recommendation is not to go mad with combinations of beans at first, as this enables you to manage quantities and take note of any particular beans that cause discomfort or uncomfortable flatulence during digestion. Pinto beans seem to set me off something wicked, if you must know!

Additives to foods, such as salt and preservatives, can also cause internal reactions such as flatulence and discomfort. If you want a fair insight into your digestive capabilities for different types of beans, always wash them before eating to reduce your chances of causing similar symptoms for other reasons.

Cooking + food prep = fun times

Since utilising more plant-based foods and introducing more plant-based proteins such as beans, pulses, and grains—I realised that my meals had a much more vibrant feel to them than ever before. My gut feeling told me that the food I was eating had life to it.

Rather than the dull colour of meat with a side of something, almost every meal was starting to look like a rainbow. I would often imagine the two dishes, meat and plant, side by side to compare them properly. It was one of the most blatant juxtapositions possible. Completely yin and yang.

I used to prep and cook my food every few days purely for health benefits—definitely not for enjoyment! Let's be honest, handling raw meat isn't exactly a laugh, is it? What got me through it was the after-effect of having ready-made, healthier options available in times of need. That was more appealing than having to settle for a more expensive, less healthy selection on the go. These days, the benefits of food prep were amplified, and the cooking part wasn't that bad either, as I didn't have to handle lifeless things!

Before the later parts of this journey, I had reached a level of creativity with my meat and animal product dishes, where I'd become comfortable with my routine and would settle on a dish mainly because it would "do the job". Statistics say that the average meat eater consumes the same 10 dishes a week for the majority of their life. Clearly it wasn't just me who had got to this sorry stage! I'm not exactly Gordon Ramsey, but I saw that there genuinely was a case to help people develop more variety in their nutrition, and this was a good start.

"Carbs make you fat"

In 2010, a professor of human nutrition wanted to prove that fat loss and gain are always a result of calories in vs. calories out, and that a caloric deficit will always cause a person to lose fat—no matter what food sources their calories come from. The study was aptly named "The Twinkie Diet".

The professor went on a 10-week diet that mostly comprised junk foods such as Twinkies (a sponge cake with cream filling), Doritos, Oreos, sugary cereals, and foods known to be highly-processed, lacking in nutritional value, loaded with sugar, high in fat, and that contain trans-fat, among other bad traits. He created a daily deficit of around 800kcal, going from eating 2600kcal per day (his estimated maintenance level) to around 1800kcal.

By the end of the study, the professor had lost 27lbs (12.2kg/1.9st). Reports state that his body fat percentage went from 33% to 25% and his BMI went from 29 to 25, essentially putting it in the "normal" range.

The Twinkie Diet pretty much proved that caloric deficit was the sole cause of fat loss. It wasn't necessarily down to the quality, but more so the quantity of foods. If the professor had wanted to gain weight, he would have done this by creating a caloric surplus instead. Even if these calories had come from healthy, plant-based foods, the excess calories would have been stored in some form in the body (often as body fat), resulting in weight gain.

Although carbs are often targeted as being the main contributor of fat gain, not all carbs are equal. All carbs are considered as 4 calories per 1g; however, for me, carb-laden junk foods and soft drinks don't come into the same category as nutritionally-dense, carb-laden plant-based foods such as fruits and veg. The former are undoubtedly one of the biggest contributors to excess calories. The latter typically contain essential nutrients for optimal body function and fibre to aid in feeling fuller for longer, which in theory means you will eat less.

- Higher levels of carbohydrate per gram are associated with processed or refined foods made from plants, including sweets, sugar, honey, soft drinks, white bread, crackers, biscuits, jam, fruit products, white pasta, and breakfast cereals. This group is often referred to as "simple carbs".
- Lower amounts of carbohydrate per gram are associated with plant-based foods, including beans, potatoes, wholegrain bread, wholegrain pasta, rice, vegetables, and unrefined fruit. This group is often referred to as "complex carbs" and usually contain more fibre than "simple carbs".

Eliminating carbs as a food group means losing essential micronutrients and dietary fibre found in fruits, vegetables, beans, legumes, and grains—ultimately inhibiting optimal bodily function. The other shame is that a forced reduction in carbs can lead to a forced increase in fat and protein consumed via animal products to account for total calorie intake, meaning increased consumption of saturated fat, cholesterol, and sodium.

It's very easy to pin the tail on the carb donkey to explain why you or someone else may be fat. As such, low-carb diets are often touted as the so-called "solution" for this. But beyond the obvious fact that you or they have been in a caloric surplus for an extended period, the real cause is habitual behaviours over an extended duration. The bigger picture is unhealthy habits and a not-so-thought-out approach to achieving optimal health.

There are many studies demonstrating that refined sugar is addictive, with the media even debating whether it's as addictive as cocaine! Addictions seem to drive irrational behaviour, and in the context of food this could mean overeating and binging, which would therefore lead to weight gain.

In very general terms, the findings up to this point appear to consistently favour the overall equation of calories in vs. calories out when it comes to weight gain and loss. Not exclusively carbs in, carbs out.

Low-carb diets may help with weight loss for the same reasons as dropping animal products. It's essentially a restricted eating pattern, and if you're not replacing your calories from carbs with anything else, then you're consuming less calories overall. And yes, the quality of not only the carbohydrates, but all food would seem to affect weight gain, as this could mean more rational behaviours surrounding food choices including resisting the urge to overeat.

The final three things I stopped eating

My mostly vegan diet was well under way and the majority of my foods had become plant-based. That being said, I was still comfortable eating a few foods that wouldn't be suitable in the next stage and consuming animal products on a daily basis! The final three things I was eating were:

- An omelette loaded with salad once a week.
- Vegetable pizza twice a week.
- Whey protein flapjacks twice a day.

I ate the omelette every Sunday morning like clockwork (though without cheese). It was like the fish finger Friday thing all over again! When it came to pizza, you might be thinking: "What happened to pizza without the cheese?!" Well, I'd bend the rules if it was frozen pizza!

While I was conscious of bending the rules with pizza and omelette, I didn't have the same feeling about whey protein flapjacks. They had been my "get out of jail card" for a long time. I kept boxes at home and in the car for times of need, like between sessions and pre/post training. I loved them because they were so filling, but without the bloat. And they were handily convenient on the go, as they came out of a packet and didn't require a fork.

Yet, for all of their practical benefits, when I looked at the ingredients list, they didn't seem all that suitable. The ingredients were unpronounceable. They were processed and I knew it. The oats softened the blow a little though, and I suppose you could say they were the best of a bad bunch compared to other protein bars. However, the ingredients always freaked me out a bit, so I tended to do the dishonourable thing and not look too often!

Looking back now, it's clear that I was able to consume two of these a day—even at this stage when my conscience was telling me otherwise—was due to disassociation with the dairy process. A whey protein flapjack appears so harmless on the surface and a million miles away from the process of obtaining its ingredients. Lovely, captivating, shiny packaging saying "high in protein", "chocolate flavoured", "slow release carbohydrates", "low in sugar". You name it, it was every health-wannabe person's dream!

I know that "bending the rules" sounds silly considering the bigger picture, but it's what went through my mind when I was eating something that contained animal products. It was a way of justifying to myself that it was okay to eat these foods from time to time. Even looking back now, it was okay, because this stage was 'mostly vegan' to serve an amazing purpose on the journey! If it had been the 'vegan' stage, then of course these foods wouldn't have been suitable.

Having gone through each stage so naturally up to this point and experienced great success with my health, it was only fair to keep the process consistent and gradually ease myself into a new routine. At least this way, the whole vegan thing didn't seem so extreme.

"Veganism is too extreme"

Classically, vegans who come across as too extreme according to mainstream society aren't those who just eat a vegan diet, but those who eat a vegan diet and protest for animal rights or partake in animal liberation. People who make noise against "the norm", and so are seen as a nuisance.

From my education up to now, I can empathise with the animal rights protestors, and in many cases, I believe what they're doing is for a good cause. But the majority of society won't unless they research and "get it" for themselves.

I've never been to a protest or taken part in animal liberation, because it's not in my personality to get involved in confrontation. This doesn't make me any less of a vegan though, does it? I'm just doing my thing! The perceived extreme part of becoming a vegan by protesting or animal liberation isn't quite the rites of passage it's made out to be. Like an initiation ceremony. Of course I'm only one person, but it shows this misconception is flawed because not all vegans are the same.

Just like "the diet", "the lifestyle" isn't a set-in-stone representation of how everyone will or should act on their beliefs on a subject. You get to decide how you let your beliefs show outside the diet and how it drives your decisions.

Yes, it's true that some people show their beliefs in a more "extreme" manner than others. However, just because you may be eating a more (or fully) plant-based diet, it doesn't necessarily mean you're automatically going to take on one of the more extreme add-ons of the diet.

Higher standards of health and wellbeing

I was on the brink of a fully plant-based diet. For the first time during this stage, I felt 100% that it could be done. I truly believed that all animal products were unnecessary in day-to-day life. Alongside this surge in clarity and motivation, I'd also been very good in the back end, researching regularly. And food prep had been a breeze lately, especially with the introduction of beans, pulses, and grains to salads, stews, and curries.

I had just completed a 3-day stint of absolutely no animal products in my system (for the first time in my life might I add), and I was experiencing health benefits I had never felt before. I felt incredible. This had a lot to do with the decisions behind my food choices:

- Generally high fibre content = fuller for longer.
- Generally lower G.I = foods absorbed into the bloodstream slower.
- Generally higher micronutrient content = nutrient requirements met.

After gradually phasing out animal products and three days on a fully plant-based diet, the benefits I experienced were:

- Better sleep: I rarely stirred during my sleep (if at all), was able to wake up better, and was more alert throughout the entire day.
- Improved energy levels overall: Back when I used to eat a lot of meat, I had a midday lull where I would have to fight the urge to nap. Now, I had a spring in my step all day (most days) and stopped experiencing a slump.
- Improved concentration and focus: My writing productivity improved tenfold. My concentration and focus in sessions was more attentive than ever.
- Much more mindful, patient, and calm: I was able to think more clearly about a lot of life-related things. I felt calmer, and had a lot more patience for just about everything.

I suppose it could be called more "mindful". This also went for the little things, such as being out driving.

- Improved fitness levels: I could exert myself a lot more than ever before. I seemed to sweat a lot less too. And I was walking faster, well over the average 3mph walking speed of a human.

- Smelling better: As reliably informed by my nearest and dearest.

- Improved digestion: I'll keep it short and sweet—my digestion felt great.

"Vegans have a higher chance of getting ill than any other diet"

Without having to be a doctor, it's intuitively known by all to avoid picking up an injury, infection, or leading an unhealthy lifestyle for an extended period. These things can all make you ill, and may lead to an earlier grave.

There are other factors that cause illness besides diet, for example, hereditary genetic conditions or a change in gene makeup, and these things are also involved in common illnesses. However, for the most part, people do what they can to avoid illness when it's in their control, such as getting sufficient sleep and not going wild every day like they might at the weekend!

The belief that malnutrition and illness are inevitable if you follow a plant-based diet is focused more on specific deficiencies in vitamins and minerals and their associated problems. Mainstream knowledge of these particular deficiencies is often where this belief comes from. Strangely, people worry more about the vegan diet than the illnesses linked to their own diet.

When talking about this misconception, people point to certain nutrients as being "lacking". Deficiencies in these areas lead to various health risks, but I've only included the most well-known here. So, let's look at some plant-based sources of these nutrients:

Protein = no muscle and overall weakness.

Soy beans, black beans, and most types of beans, lentils, protein powders such as pea, rice or soy, hemp seeds, chia seeds, pumpkin seeds, spirulina, peanuts, most types of nuts and nut butters, quinoa, seitan, tempeh, and tofu.

Vitamin B6 = damage to the nervous system.

Many whole grain and fortified cereals, pistachios, sage, paprika, parsley, chilli powder, chives, basil, wheatgerm, jackfruit, amaranth, oregano, dried and shiitake mushrooms.

Vitamin B12 = damage to the nervous system.

Fortified soy products, fortified plant-based milks, breakfast cereals, and yeast extract spread.

Calcium = weak bones.

Unhulled sesame seeds, tahini, almonds, tofu, collard greens, basil, thyme and many other herbs, molasses, dandelion greens, black eyed peas, seaweed, rocket, kale, watercress, spinach, hazelnuts, pak choi, okra, sunflower seeds, broccoli, oranges and raw agave.

Vitamin D = osteoporosis.

Fortified plant-based milk and cereal grains, alfalfa, mushrooms—most, if not all types. And the sun, but you can't eat that!

Iron = anaemia.

Thyme, basil, cumin and many other herbs, soy beans, most types of beans, molasses, lentils, chickpeas, spinach, tofu, cashew nuts, chia seeds, flaxseed, hemp seeds, pumpkin seeds, kale, dried apricots, dried figs, raisins, quinoa, amaranth, spirulina, soy protein isolate, and fortified breakfast cereal.

Omega-3 = mental function and depression.

Flax oil, flaxseeds, pumpkin seeds, hemp seeds, and chia seeds.

Other plant-based foods that have notable health benefits include: Berries, wholegrains, dark leafy greens, cruciferous vegetables, and herbal teas.

By including these plant-based sources in your diet, you can ensure you don't become deficient, or improve the situation if you're already deficient.

Ultimately, it doesn't matter if your nutritional preferences gain you a potentially unwanted title in society, such as "vegan" or "vegetarian", because the bottom line is: if you don't eat enough of the right foods, you will become deficient in certain nutrients, whether you eat meat or not. Simple as.

This is why you see so many meat eaters still getting ill. Yet nobody questions whether a meat eater's illness is related to certain deficiencies in their diet. People just assume that it's "bad luck" when meat eaters get ill. But when a vegan or vegetarian gets ill—it's deemed to be because of their diet.

I'm not even joking. At some point, a bug was doing the rounds in my area. Everyone was off sick from work, and it had people bed-bound. I rarely get sick, but this time I caught a chest infection and couldn't work. Someone I knew caught the bug two weeks before I did. Yet they asked me, "Do you think you got it because you don't eat meat?" This person ate meat, supplements, and animal products on a daily basis, and they'd had the bug for two weeks. Yet, they were speculating that my diet was the cause of my illness. We had the same illness. The irony was, I shook off the bug after two weeks and was back to full speed, while they had it for another two weeks!

It's worth noting that if someone adopts a plant-based diet with a thought-out approach to nutrition—one that provides sufficient intake of all of the nutrients, then it actually appears to provide many health benefits. This includes a reduced risk of type 2 diabetes, high blood pressure, obesity, and heart disease. On the contrary to the misconception, vegans were shown to have lower blood pressure, lower BMI, and lower cholesterol.

In some studies, a plant-based diet was also associated with a significant reduction in cancer risk. Cancer-protective factors associated with the diet include the increased consumption of fruits, vegetables, plant-based proteins including soy, and a lower BMI.

Likewise, it's thought that excess body weight contributes to one in five cancer-related deaths in the U.S., and that around 20% of all cancers diagnosed there are related to high body fat, lack of physical inactivity, excess alcohol consumption, and/or poor nutrition.

Genetic conditions aside, a fruitful combination of due diligence, knowledge, and application in nutrition undoubtedly have the most influence in whether someone gets ill or not. If someone doesn't think out their diet and nutrition, then whatever their "title", they're increasing their chances of getting ill.

It's what's on the inside that counts

On the inside, I felt like a zillion dollars, my genuine best-ever self. But on the outside, I wasn't looking my so-called "best". It turned out that writing a book and not training very often was catching up with me. My goals had changed completely since embarking on this journey, and over time, my physique had started to reflect this change for all to see... and comment on!

When my body first started changing, the majority decision was that I looked better, "sickeningly healthy." But this time, people didn't seem so sure. If anyone instigated a conversation with me about my appearance, I got the vibe from their body language and tone that they didn't agree with how I looked now. I was apparently "looking skinny".

After checking in on my body composition, I'd lost another 3kg, bringing my total weight loss down to 10kg on this journey. I was now 85kg, and my body fat levels were around the same as before. My weight loss suggested that I had been consistently living in a caloric deficit. Although I wasn't trying to under-eat, the scales showed I had been. Despite feeling awesome, I didn't want to be in a calorie deficit for much longer.

According to some studies, nearly 65% of people who go on a crash diet to lose weight return to their pre-diet weight within three years. This shows that trying to do too much too soon isn't helpful in the long term. I wasn't on a crash diet, but I certainly didn't want to rebound the other way.

I had to face the fact that I hadn't been eating enough for my daily expenditure. I had been eating an amazingly varied array of plant-based foods... however, I hadn't taken into account that the high fibre content makes them very filling. If I didn't want to be in a caloric deficit, I needed to eat a higher volume of plant-based foods to meet my caloric requirements.

It's also worth noting that I was consuming far less calories from fat, as I had reduced animal product intake such as cheese and eggs. Fat has the highest calories of all the macronutrients, so a big chunk of my calories had gone.

Chances are that not many people will transition to a plant-based diet and start writing a book at the same time. But the key takeaway is that regardless of your nutritional preferences, if you change your goals and subsequently your lifestyle in order to reach them, you may experience a few teething problems while you work out what will give you the best results.

"Veganism is an eating disorder"

Eating disorders are characterised by an abnormal attitude towards food. One that causes someone to change their eating habits and behaviour. Someone with an eating disorder may focus excessively on their weight and shape, leading them to make unhealthy choices about food—with damaging results to their health. Their diet is seen to be ultra-restrictive in comparison to the no-holds-barred approach to food in the conventional Western diet.

The restriction aspect of eating disorders ties into the belief that a plant-based diet is also restrictive, leading people to think that they're the same.

The most common eating disorders are:

- Anorexia nervosa: When a person tries to keep their weight as low as possible, for example, by starving themselves or exercising excessively.
- Bulimia: When a person goes through periods of binge eating and is then deliberately sick or uses laxatives to control their weight.
- Binge eating disorder (BED): When a person feels compelled to over-eat large amounts of food in a short space of time.
- EDNOS: Some people, particularly those who are young, may be diagnosed with an eating disorder not otherwise specified (EDNOS). This means they have some, but not all, of the typical signs of eating disorders.

The main cause of eating disorders is commonly blamed on social pressure to be thin, with young people in particular feeling they should look a certain way. However, the causes are often more complex. An eating disorder may be associated with biological, genetic, or environmental factors combined with a particular event that triggers the disorder. There may also be other factors that maintain the illness, such as an anxiety disorder or depression.

In a study on the relationship between veganism, vegetarianism, and eating disorders, it was found that some people with eating disorders label themselves as vegetarians or vegans "so they won't have to eat." As such, the research indicates that the majority of vegetarian/vegan anorexics and bulimics chose their diets after the onset of the disease, not the other way around.

This is likely because adopting the vegetarian or vegan diet can legitimise and justify the removal of numerous foods to others—without scrutiny. Foods that are often avoided by people with eating disorders are those seen as high-fat and energy-dense, such as meat, eggs, and cheese.

Eating patterns chosen by those with eating disorders are generally far more restrictive than a mindfully healthy vegetarian or vegan diet. This is mainly due to those with eating disorders limiting their overall caloric intake—while vegetarians and vegans generally do not aim to do so. People with eating disorders may therefore also eliminate nutrient-dense, higher-fat plant-based foods such as nuts, seeds, and avocados—while vegetarians and vegans often increase their intake of these foods.

In my personal experience, I have come across many people who stated that a plant-based diet or veganism in general actually helped them overcome their eating disorder and made them healthy. That being said, it will always come down to the individual and not the diet—that old chestnut.

Animal products are literally everywhere!

When it came to buying food, I knew I had to be assertive in reading the ingredients, especially for mainstream products that looked convenient and appealing. I also had a general idea of which products were a bit shifty and which were okay using good old common sense.

However, I assumed that single-ingredient and plant-based foods were surely free from animal products. They are, right?! Wrong! In fact, when I first realised the true scope of animal products, I was eating fruit!

I'd purchased a frozen bag of 'tropical mix' from the shop, containing papaya, pineapple, mango, and coconut. Halfway through the bowl, my mouth tasted a bit "milky", as if I was eating ice cream. I checked the bag and sure enough, my taste buds weren't lying. The coconut pieces contained skimmed milk powder! I couldn't believe how unnecessary it was to put dairy in a bag of fruit. I literally felt doomed, like I couldn't escape animal products.

While I had felt bombarded with veggie options in the vegetarian stage, there were very few occasions in this stage that I came across something in the mainstream specifically marketed as vegan-friendly. It became clear that I would have to look harder. At first, it felt like I'd have to read literally everything about a product before buying it, or check for the magic "V word".

After a while, I realised this wasn't working, because many products weren't suitable for vegans or had been marketed as something else, such as dairy-free. There were also labels such as: gluten-free, non-GMO, soya-free, suitable for vegetarians, lactose-free, and no added sugars or sweeteners.

While I was getting used to everything, I found this kind of marketing very distracting. Without the 'suitable for vegans' hallmark or something similar, I wasn't sure whether items were actually vegan-friendly. I would end up not buying something if I wasn't sure, and often going hungry for peace of mind.

I truly realised at this stage that you could not trust the packet! As tedious as it may sound, I had to cross-check every product by looking through the ingredients list. This was most confusing part when I had cross-checked all the ingredients and it seemed to be vegan-friendly, yet the packet said 'suitable for vegetarians'. It left me questioning: "So is this vegan-friendly or not?!"

This confusion led me to more research, and I was shocked to find out that beyond milk powder, which was the usual culprit, there were other animal products to look out for, such as:

Carmine

Made up from crushed up beetles. Often found in foods that are coloured with a natural red dye, such as soft drinks and syrups.

Gelatin

A protein obtained mainly by boiling tendons, skin, bones, and ligaments with water, usually from pigs or cows. Found in sweets and confectionery. In plant-based foods, agar is often used in place of gelatin.

Dashi

Known as "Japanese sea stock", it can be found in many "vegetable dishes". Traditional versions often include these animal ingredients: kelp, dried bonito flakes (a type of fish), or dried baby sardines.

Castoreum

Derived from the anal glands of beavers (yummy!). Mainly used in foods and beverages as part of a substitute vanilla flavour.

Isinglass:

Gelatin from fish bladders. Sometimes found in beer, jelly, and confectionery. Not as commonly found now.

L-cysteine

An amino acid reportedly derived from human hair or poultry feathers including duck. Most commonly found in bagels, pizza, bread, and fast food restaurants that provide buns and other 'doughy' stuff.

Lactic acid

Not to be confused with what the human body produces during intense exercise! In food, it's a dairy product formed by bacteria on lactose. Found in some pickles, pickled vegetables, olives, dressings, soft drinks, fruit juice, and bread.

Omega 3

Sometimes, omega-3 from fish oils is added to products such as fruit juice and joint supplements.

After this realisation, I went straight to the ingredients list to use my better judgement. I didn't take the packaging too literally, whether it proclaimed to be vegan-friendly or not. Or even if it seemed blatantly obvious that it would be vegan-friendly, like the frozen fruit. It's safe to say that you can expect the unexpected.

"If you make a mistake and eat something you shouldn't, then you're not technically a vegan"

This misconception might sound strange, but there may come a time when you accidentally consume animal products around other people and they voice their thoughts on it! How you react to this depends on the person's tone and body language, i.e. are they being a dick about it, or genuinely interested?

In essence, the statement is true. Technically, you wouldn't be a vegan if you consumed animal products. However, if you were trying not to consume animal products and you accidentally did, then it's not true. The difference in what technically makes you a vegan is down to your due diligence. In other words, how much care do you take over your diet? It's also down to whether you perceive yourself as a "vegan" or just refer to yourself as, well, you!

Due diligence is when someone takes reasonable steps to avoid committing an offence. In business, it's when you do everything in your power to make it work. From how you treat other staff members and employees to how your actions represent the business. In a plant-based diet, due diligence means you take reasonable steps to avoid consuming animal products, as per the template of a plant-based diet. As opposed to showing zero due diligence to the template and not caring about eating animals or animal products.

Reasonable steps in this context include vetting the ingredients of what you are about to eat to ensure that everything is vegan-friendly. Every now and then, this may be obvious from the product label in the form of a vegan hallmark. But for the most part, you'll have to check the ingredients list. In 2015, a U.S. study found that less than 38% of people trust what companies say on labels. So, you wouldn't be alone if you did a little more due diligence there.

In fact, there have been many times when I had my usual high standard of due diligence, yet still found myself caught short, accidentally eating animal products. Around other people too. This is especially likely when there's no packaging. I'm talking from experience when I say that someone may feel the need to say you're not a vegan after all, or a shit one at best!

This, memorably, happened to me at a wedding. It was close to the end of the evening celebrations. Everyone was drunk as fuck. I was sober and hungry as fuck. A buffet of food suddenly appeared and it was like an oasis in the desert. It wasn't just your usual spread that came out either—it was a quirky "Sunday roast dinner themed" spread. There were roast potatoes, a gravy fountain, and what looked like deep-fried, breaded mushrooms.

My gut feeling told me to ask the servers what was in the deep-fried things, and what the potatoes had been cooked in, because you never know. But I couldn't see any servers, so I asked some random drunk people and they replied, "I think it's mushrooms". They looked like mushrooms on the inside just as much as the outside.

But, after a few potatoes and a few breaded things, I started to get a weird, thick taste in my mouth and at the bottom of my throat. It reminded me of when I accidentally ate cheese the week before in what was supposed to be a vegetable curry wrap from the supermarket. Something wasn't right.

I started to regret not asking a server. I began to ask a few more drunk people, and they all said they thought it was mushrooms. I didn't mention why I was asking or drop the "V bomb". I just made out that I was asking for the sake of asking. As if I was a breaded mushroom connoisseur or something!

But I couldn't keep eating with this unwanted nostalgic, thick coagulating lump in the back of my throat. So, I went looking for a server and asked what was in the breaded things. It turned not to be mushrooms. It was beef! Beef! I felt sick, horrified actually. As if cheese sneaking into your vegetable curry wrap and milk sneaking into your frozen fruit wasn't bad enough already... now beef was sneaking into what looked like a safe-bet breaded mushroom! At least the potatoes had been cooked in vegetable oil and not beef dripping. I learnt that lesson a few weeks back when I ate chips from a chip shop that turned out to be cooked in beef dripping.

As if I wasn't already feeling bad enough about not taking the proper due diligence to avoid meat, and feeling horrendous with a belly full of beef, I had to deal with subjective statements about my diet. We'll call it "banter".

"So does that mean you're not a vegan now?"
Me: "I never said that I was a vegan in the first place. I'm Glen."

"How long does it technically take for you to become a vegan again now that you've eaten beef?"
Supposedly there is a timeframe on how long it takes for you to become a vegan after eating something that isn't vegan-friendly?

"Are you going to go and make yourself sick?"
Everyone thought this was the solution and I'd suddenly be a vegan again.

"You might as well eat more seeing as you already have— I won't tell anyone!"
This is an example of the "fuck it" attitude. It happens with food, and generally when people make a mistake. They see it like this: you've already fucked up, so you may as well fuck up some more! And then some.

"I don't see what the problem is, eating beef is normal..."
As the person stating this genuinely didn't show any remorse, I just diffused the situation there and then. My simple reply was: "Same here actually".

You can see from this that the perception of a vegan diet from the general public (albeit drunk) is that there are rules in how and when the diet kicks in based on timeframes. There's also an element of fascination and imagination in such statements. How you react to this is what makes it an issue or not.

Frozen meat- and fish-based alternatives

There was never a time on this journey when I craved meat or thought to myself: "I'd love to eat a burger right now." That being said, I was looking for some new meal ideas that were practical to make and suitable for this stage.

I was eating a lot of whole foods, big hearty meals, and what some people would consider "clean". But I needed that little bit of "naughty" in my diet, something that wasn't sweet or fresh. I also wanted something lazy, in that it could cook itself, for example, as a weekend treat. Something like fish finger Fridays was obviously off the menu these days, but that's not to say I wouldn't be able to get veggie or vegan alternatives to them if I looked.

To me, veggie sausages and veggie burgers didn't sound so bad in comparison to veggie fish. So, I thought that if I was going to give these meat/fish-based alternatives a whirl, I'd go for some that weren't fish for now. Off to my local supermarket I went in search of these frozen foods. I found some that were suitable for vegans, looked edible, and didn't even taste too bad. Dare I say it, they actually tasted good?

What freaked me out was how they actually looked and tasted just like meat. So much so that the first time I tried them, I felt uncomfortable. In fact, I had to check the packet again to make sure I hadn't accidentally picked up real meat. For me, it didn't make any sense to want to eat a plant-based diet yet still eat things that resembled an animal.

Then I tried bean-style varieties of burgers, sausages, and fish fingers. They were less of a meat replica, and in the beginning, they were a lot tastier. The thought of eating meat, or even something that looked like it, made me feel queasy. So the bean versions were more suitable for me at this stage.

Overall, I wouldn't recommend that you rely on these kind of foods altogether, as the mainstream versions aren't exactly healthy. They often contain excess oil, salt, and sugars. However, it's nice from time to time to have an easy option when you fancy being lazy.

From my findings, it was clear that these foods weren't going to be the most healthy for me. What's more, a lot of them contained animal products such as cheese, milk, or eggs. Most of them are marketed at the more in-demand veggie market than the vegan market. It's good to be aware of this if you go looking for meat-based alternatives at this stage.

Based on my research, it seemed that many people use meat-based alternatives to help them transition more smoothly to a plant-based diet, because they can keep their meals looking the same, or near enough. However, this is something that people often try at the beginning of the journey while they phase out meat. Trust me to do it backwards!

"I think I could go vegan, but I couldn't give up cheese because I'm addicted"

Sometimes, people reach a stage where change is needed, but they realise they love something too much to give it up. This is when the "fuck it" attitude can creep in. For example, thinking "If I can't give up cheese, then I may as well not give up anything." Or even try to take on a plant-based diet.

However, just because someone can't give up cheese, or bacon, or chocolate, it doesn't mean this is the case for everyone trying to move on to a plant-based diet. So, if you know of or have heard of someone who attempted it but loved cheese too much, that's just them. It might be different for you.

It is true that, like bacon and most other fatty foods containing animal products, cheese is said to be highly addictive. So much so that the mainstream say it triggers the same part of brain as hard drugs like cocaine and heroin! Cheese = dairy crack? Jheeze.

Let's look at the actual science. Some studies suggest that cheese addiction is particularly potent because it contains casein (also found in cow's milk). When casein breaks down in the stomach, it produces peptide and casomorphin, a substance present in all dairy products. This substance is thought to trigger the brain's opioid receptors, which are linked to addiction.

One study found that processed foods were linked to addictive behaviour more than unprocessed foods, with fatty foods being the most addictive. The top-ranking foods on the addiction scale also often contained cheese. Pizzas, cheeseburgers, and just cheese featured in the top 10. Interestingly, the top 10 least-addictive foods were mostly whole, plant-based, and unprocessed. Cucumbers, carrots, and beans made the top three.

It's important to remember that processed foods are usually engineered to be "hyper-palatable". Meaning they have been made to taste super good and be more tempting than unprocessed foods. Think about the marketing that comes with these types of food, pizzas, burgers, and so on. Do you ever see cucumber being marketed like this?!

"Being tasty" sounds like a good thing; however, addictive-like eating behaviour involves a lot more than just a lack of willpower. There are said to be biochemical reasons why some people lose control over their consumption, and potentially their health.

Eating processed food such as cheese releases massive amounts of feel-good chemicals compared to unprocessed foods. This yields a much more powerful "reward" in the brain. Doing drugs such as cocaine or eating too much junk food gradually overload the so-called "pleasure centres" in the brain. Eventually, these pleasure centres crash. Then, achieving the same pleasure or even just feeling normal requires an increase in the amount of drug or food.

Food addiction and addictive-like eating behaviours are serious problems that certain foods are more likely to trigger. You could take this as another reason to base your diet mostly on whole, plant-based, single-ingredient foods. These foods release an appropriate amount of feel-good chemicals in the brain to make up for satiety, while also ensuring you don't overeat.

No food prep = so much panic!

It was the weekend and I had a lot of sessions to do. Two of my clients had similar goals. They were both relatively new runners training for an upcoming adventure run. As a result, I was running with them in their sessions to work through some coaching points. Obviously, to run twice in the same day, I needed to be well-fed to keep my energy levels up. You'd think that having suitable, high-energy food prepped would be the most logical approach. But no, I flopped!

When I woke up that day, I realised the cupboards were pretty bare. Instead of salvaging everything in there to get through the day, I shrugged it off with an "it'll be fine" kind of attitude. My theory was I could get something on the go, even though it wouldn't be as high-quality as something prepared at home. I thought, what's the worst that could happen?

After a few sessions and a fair run with my first running client, I was ravenous! En route to my next client and in a bit of a rush, I popped into an express supermarket. At first, I was confident there would be something suitable, since vegan food is trending in the mainstream and organic food sales are at an all-time high.

However, in the go-to places for snacks, I began to get frustrated. It turned out there was nothing I could eat unless I went "junk food veggie" with a crappy cheese or egg sandwich. Although officially still in the "mostly vegan" stage, I was really trying to set myself up for the future. By making these decisions now, I'd know the answers for later in the journey.

Panic stations set in. I couldn't find a single balanced meal that was suitable for vegans. The irony was, even the readymade superfood salads contained meat, fish, or an animal product lathered over it in the form of dressing. In desperation, after bouncing from aisle to aisle, I realised the only practical food choice was fruit! Now, there's nothing wrong with fruit, but I was being stubborn at my limited choice in times of need. Even the nuts there were salted or roasted, not in their natural form. For the first time, the thought crossed my mind, being on a plant-based diet is shit!

In a strop, I decided not to settle for fruit. My attempt to leave the store was delayed though, as my eyes rested on a full-size French bread stick strategically placed by the door. Hunger had truly got the better of me, because I saw this big, white baguette as my saviour! I bought it, and weirdly nothing else to go with it. Before reaching my car, I'd already started tucking into it. With no sauce or anything. By the time I arrived at the client's, I had eaten the whole thing!

My perceived starvation and stubbornness over the contrast of choice between a "normal" diet and a plant-based diet had me wolfing down what must have been a metre of French bread in one sitting! This may be a tad melodramatic, but I felt quite emotional about it. Plus, a bit anxious that I was in a hot car, about to go for another run, with a whole French stick sitting uncomfortably in my belly! The entire situation was chaotic and completely out of character. It was all rush, rush, rush. As you can imagine, I didn't feel so great running after that! Though I put on a brave face for my client.

Later that day, my digestive system was shot, and most of the following day too. Never before had I desired to eat a whole French stick with nothing on it, and this probably goes for most people! All in all, it was a massive learning curve, a lesson in preparation. It taught me so much about what it would be like moving to the next stage. After that, I made sure to ever let myself get so ravenous and have plenty of snacks on hand, such as:

- Nuts: Mixed nuts, most varieties, all of the time.
- Seeds: Pumpkin seeds, sunflower seeds.
- Fruit: Bananas, pears, apples, kiwis (generally non-messy fruits)!

- Dried fruit: Dates, prunes, raisins, apricots.
- Natural energy bars: Vegan-friendly.

"I can't be bothered to cook and prep food because it's boring"

There are many reasons why prepping food in advance will serve you better than scrambling something together on the go and hoping for the best! First, you'll probably eat healthier than you would at the last minute, or at least be more mindful of your goals. Second, you'll probably spend less money by buying more food in bulk. Plus, having food ready means less stress when you're starving, low on time, and can't find a suitable option on the go.

Could you be doing something more fun and exhilarating with your time rather than prepping your food? Of course you could! Though some foodies might disagree. It's a personal thing whether you enjoy food prep or not.

At the beginning, it might feel a bit shit. You may be tentatively following recipes step by step. Scared to get one ingredient wrong. Or you may just throw a load of healthy, plant-based food in a bowl and cross your fingers. Without even knowing their individual flavours and nutritional value.

Interestingly, you wouldn't be the only one who feels this way. A study in the UK of 2,000 adults found that lack of time and confidence about nutrition plays havoc with the average person's meal plans. Around 60% of UK residents eat the same dishes week after week. It was also found that 1 in 4 adults cook the same meal on the same day every week and even have a strict rota in place for nearly 4 years. Around 13% of them eat the same thing on the same day for 10 years or more! No wonder why people think food prep is boring and are excited by random food on the go.

One study examined the eating and cooking habits of 4,000 UK households from 1980 to 2012 and found that people spend around 34 minutes preparing evening meals compared to a full hour in 1980. Cooking time has reduced by almost a minute a year on average. And sandwiches have become the most commonly eaten "meal" over the course of the day.

With this in mind, it's no wonder why so many people take a shortcut and eat the most convenient things. This is reflected in the top three most popular evening meals in the UK, all takeaways: Indian, Chinese, and pizza.

Food prep is a fucker, because you have to do something proactive in your free time! But if you can focus on what you'll get back from these short blocks of time, then it's not the hardest thing in the world. If you start to do this, then you'll see the value in it. You'll do it regardless of your feelings towards it.

You'll definitely see the value in it if you're heading towards a fully plant-based diet and get caught short on the go, where you have to settle for anything vegan-friendly. Healthy or not.

If you're like me, then you'll savour the time and make it feel more productive and rewarding. Like listening to audiobooks, podcasts, or music to jazz up the time while cooking if you find it boring.

Eating out

During this stage, I hadn't really eaten out. Then, one of my family members suggested we go a restaurant to celebrate a family birthday. There were three of us going, including me. After a great experience at a particular restaurant, one family member suggested we go there. We'll call her Doris.

Doris is lactose-intolerant and avoids all dairy products but eats meat every now and then. She highly recommended the place as she'd been impressed with their quality of food. She believed she was familiar with their selection of dairy-free meals and was certain they had a good selection of vegan food on their diverse menu. So, it was a no-brainer to go there really.

I liked the look of the vegetarian breakfast, which had spinach, tomatoes, mushroom, baked beans, sourdough bread, "vegetarian" sausages, and eggs. As you can imagine, the first thing I questioned was the validity of the vegetarian sausages. Did this mean they were actually vegetarian? Or was it another marketing ploy for the masses as they were actually vegan?

Doris said she'd had the meal before and it was nice. I asked whether the sausages contained cheese, as many veggie sausages and meat-free alternatives do. She confidently said no. She said she would know because she didn't have any problems with her digestion after eating them previously.

So, when the waitress came over to take our order, I had faith in Doris and didn't ask about the sausages. I replaced the eggs with avocado and was happy with my choice. We all enjoyed the meal, had an espresso for dessert, and off we went happily ever after.

After the meal, there was nothing irregular going on with my body, but my intuition told me there was cheese in the sausages. I called the restaurant and they explained that the fucking sausages aren't suitable for vegans, as they contain cheese!

I didn't cry about it, but I did decide to learn a lesson from it, so I'd never make the same mistake again. I trusted Doris—she is family after all. But after this, I would always confidently ask the server no matter how silly the question seemed... and I wouldn't trust my family to know the answers again!

From speaking to people, one of the biggest concerns about following a plant-based diet (even if they wanted to try it) is inconvenience and feeling like they are poking their neck out of line in asking for a vegan option. When you're starting out on a plant-based diet, you may feel like the odds are against you in terms of choice. Especially when eating out in restaurants.

It's a shame that most meals in restaurants don't come with information about the ingredients, so you could be sure without having to ask. Maybe this will be the case one day, but we're not there yet. In the meantime, I hope you use my bad experiences to identify where you need to be assertive for your benefit.

They say "ignorance is bliss", but pretending to be so ignorant towards something that clearly means a lot to you can be detrimental to your wellbeing. Always remember that you have a right to know what you're eating—just the same as everyone else does.

"If you make a bit of a scene at a restaurant, the waiter will do something to your meal"

We've all been there. You're in a restaurant. Waiting on your food. Eventually it comes out and it's not what you ordered. Or worse, it tastes dodgy! Next, you're calling for the server's attention. In the back of your mind, you're thinking that you better tread carefully in explaining it to the server. Or something unwelcome and strictly off-menu might be added to your meal.

When you start working towards your plant-based diet, you have to tweak things a little until they become natural and you no longer feel like you're adjusting things. Doing this when eating out can be a bit awkward at first. So, your first step to success is getting over the belief that you're being a pain in the arse to accommodate your "weird" needs. You need to grow in confidence here.

The next step is getting over the reaction of the server. You don't need to go into detail and start banging on about your life story, your reasons for adopting a plant-based diet, and why you want to change something on the menu. If things go a little preachy, then your meal might not go so peachy! Just ask whether they can accommodate a particular request for you and see what they come back with. If they ask you a little more, or guess that you're a vegan, then just say "yeah". Just like you would if you had a food allergy.

In the UK, it's estimated that 1-2% of adults and 5-8% of children have a food allergy. That's around 2 million people, and this doesn't include food intolerances. Common allergies include cow's milk, peanuts, eggs, shellfish, tree nuts, wheat, rice, and fruit. The most common allergies vary depending on location. Allergies are often a result of genetics and are hereditary.

Symptoms of allergies include itchiness, tongue swelling, vomiting, diarrhoea, hives, trouble breathing, or low blood pressure. These typically occur within minutes up to several hours after exposure. When the symptoms are severe, it's known as anaphylaxis. This is when the body has become hypersensitive.

When it comes to food allergies, not only is the individual likely to be assertive about their condition, but those who care for the person are too. Friends and family members often speak up on the person's behalf. The attitude about allergies is: the server needs to know. And the restaurant will cater for the allergy as best they can. Having a negative reaction isn't great publicity!

A study in the U.S. found that just 2% of people always make reservations to eat at restaurants, while 35% never make restaurant reservations. Since making the transition to a plant-based diet, being in the 2% every time I go out to eat is far better! It's given me so much peace of mind to reserve and discuss my dietary needs upfront to see whether they can be met.

Most restaurants aim to please when you discuss your plant-based diet. However, there may be some places that just don't get it. Particularly if you're having this conversation in person. In these cases, be nice, jovial, and empathetic! Don't be condescending and expect them to know everything your diet entails. In these times, you need to be composed, because you want the server on your side, and this is why...

- A U.S. survey found that 80% of 438 food service employees admitted to "harmless activities" like making fun of a difficult customer behind their back or lying to a customer. If you want to uphold your plant-based diet standards when you're out, then you need the server to tell you the truth.

- If your service is a little slower than usual, it could be on purpose, because 65% admitted to taking their time if they didn't like a customer.
- The bad news is that 6% admitted to contaminating food. A pretty horrific thought. The good news is that it's only 6%.

There are many surveys that go into the finer details of servers sabotaging people's restaurant experiences. However, none of this points significantly to vegans being the victim. The main point seems to be whether you're a dick to the server first, they're having a bad day, or they're a bit of a dick naturally.

MOSTLY VEGAN summary

Set rules you can stick to.

Creating simple rules that you truly believe you can be consistent with will create long-term habits. If it's something as blatant as only eating chocolate if it's vegan-friendly, then do it.

Make beans, pulses, and grains work for you.

Grains can be treated like beans and pulses, as they fit easily into your diet and bump up your micronutrients. Go for variety, and opt for wholegrain, low G.I varieties when you're sedentary to avoid hunger and a carb coma!

Eat more salad!

Prep your salad daily if you prefer maximum freshness, or every other day to save time. Include lots of things that you enjoy, but also many things that you know you should be eating more of (make healthy choices)!

Maximise the potential of designated cooking time.

Learn to make food prep more interesting. Listen to upbeat music or even a motivational audiobook/podcast. Make it feel like you're unwinding and not simply being controlled by your food. You may even learn something!

Bend the rules every now and then.

Allow yourself to make mistakes and don't put too much pressure on yourself initially. Think long term, as any corners you cut at this stage can and will be improved over time, as you gain experience and knowledge.

Drop the ego (outside) and think health (inside).

"Beauty" comes and goes with trends, so opinions on what is and isn't beautiful will change. Plus, what you feel on the inside will show on the outside. And being healthy on the inside will never go out of fashion.

Don't trust the packaging... EVER!

Be assertive when reading food packaging. It may be suitable for vegans without specifically highlighting this. Take the time to research other USPs (such as dairy-free) and always check the ingredients list to be double-sure.

Don't be afraid to break tradition to suit you better.

Wanting to alter your meal slightly is perfectly acceptable in this modern era, where we are often spoilt for choice. "Traditional" meals are based on their own time when they were created. So, create your own for these times.

Take a "food prep" state of mind the night before.

In the nicest possible way, take control of your nutrition because nobody is going to do it for you! Look at your upcoming schedule and prepare your nutrition accordingly so you have time to prepare your food in advance.

Never let yourself get ravenous.

To avoid eating anything and everything and potentially ruining your plant-based diet, keep yourself satisfied throughout the day with healthy snacks between meals. Crunchy foods such as carrots, celery, and cucumbers are convenient and filling.

Restaurants want to keep their customers happy.

As a customer, you have the power! Pluck up the courage to discuss your needs in advance (by calling to book) or at the restaurant. As the old saying goes, you don't ask, you don't get.

Stage Five
VEGAN

Embracing it

Taking on the title of "vegan" seemed a bit cringey at the beginning. I just wanted to be "Glen John Jones". The bloke who privately changed his diet to suit his goals, then went about his own business without having to declare it to the rest of society. For a while, I got a bit of stick from friends and family.

"Why do you always need to take things to the extreme?"
"You're going to lose your body that you've worked so hard for!"
"You're not going to turn into an annoying prick now, are you?"
"You're going to get ill and end up in hospital!"

However, it wasn't long before all of these people got on board. Especially when they realised that none of these concerns materialised. In fact, once they had got all of their subjective beliefs off their chests, they literally couldn't do enough for me and were more concerned than I was about upholding my diet and not eating food that contained animal products.

"Are you sure that's going to be okay for you?"
"I can get you something else if it's not good enough."
"I've been researching vegan-friendly recipes for the next time we get together for dinner. Some of them look really nice actually!"
"I've seen that there's a vegan food festival coming up soon in London and I wondered if you wanted to go together?"

I realised that my original epiphany about the vegan diet was wrong. That being, the longer I utilised it, the more people would move away from me because the majority of people in society are prejudiced against it. I had worried that I would become isolated and left out.

Surprisingly, the opposite turned out to be true. It seemed like more people were actually drawn towards me, purely out of interest. It may sound like I was lapping up the attention and enjoying it! The truth is though that I still only wanted to be that bloke "Glen John Jones". Not "Glen John Jones, the vegan".

Embracing the title definitely helped to smooth things over in the long term, as it eventually became "normal" to those around me. So much so that they would relish catering to my needs! In fact, they even began to tweak their own diet in my presence to be more vegan-friendly too. Not that I needed them too, but they wanted to. Who would have thought it?

"How do you know whether someone is vegan? They tell you"

I won't lie to you—there are people who happen to be vegan and who are also fucking annoying! That said, I know more annoying meat eaters than annoying vegans. Probably because there are more meat eaters overall.

This misconception is a kickback from all the annoying vegans of the past who felt the need to speak more than listen. In particular, speak more about themselves. Name-dropping the "V word" without being asked or without it being relevant to the conversation.

This misconception exists because when some vegans feel the urge to drop the "V word", it can be out of context to the rest of the conversation. This makes it appear like a cry for attention, a bit show-offy, or obsessive over being a vegan. For non-vegans, this proves their misconception to be right.

Non-vegan: So, I was going for a life-changing job interview the other day and...

Vegan butts in: That's really fascinating, did I ever tell you about this really cool vegan-friendly cafe I've just found on the internet?

Non-vegan: Oh, no you didn't, but anyway, everything was going well at this life-changing interview and then...

Vegan butts in again: Yeah, they do loads of smoothies and stuff and it's like so totes cool because everyone in there is vegan and vegans are the best... and so on.

It doesn't have to be like that though. I recently started coaching a new client who I'd known for a couple of years, along with her partner. She explained what they both eat and their aims. Funnily enough, she said she would one day like to take on a plant-based diet, having seen a few documentaries. But she didn't know how to and didn't think it was possible in modern society.

At this point, she had opened the conversation, so I dropped the "V word": "Not sure if you knew already, but I've been on a plant-based diet for a while now, so I can 100% vouch for you that it is possible."

She said, "No way! I would never have guessed. How do you feel?"

I replied: "Not just saying this, but I feel incredible. Best I've ever felt. Mentally, physically, etc. If you ever want to know more, we could cover it another time."

The conversation then briefly went into nutrient deficiency (especially protein), convenience, and goals. I kept it short and sweet, then pretty much changed the subject, making it out to not be such a big deal. Then we got on with the training session.

Because I'd let the conversation come to me, the end result was that she felt inspired. If I gone to her and dropped the "V word" out of context or not at the right moment, then it wouldn't have made such a good impression in her eyes. Instead, it would have seemed like I was trying to make an impression and get attention. The right moment in this instance was when she mentioned it first and effectively "qualified" for me to open up about my own experience.

Naturally caring more for the environment

When I started caring more for the environment, my concern was that I may be on the road to tying myself to a tree at a protest! The word "enlightenment" springs to mind. I try not to sound as "out there" and hippy as the word implies, but the truth is that it's a great word to describe the process of this plant-based journey and what you go through from start to finish.

The word enlightenment is linked to concepts such as: understanding, insight, education, learning, knowledge, awareness, information, wisdom, instruction, teaching, light, awakening, woke, culture, sophistication, advancement, and development.

Prior to starting my own transition, I wouldn't litter. I'd shower instead of taking baths. I'd walk as much as I could rather than driving. Partly because I enjoy walking, but also because it's beneficial environmentally, economically, and health-wise. The only reason I don't cycle is because I live just outside London, where the roads are unsafe and chaotic.

Without having to do any research on what's beneficial for the environment, these actions are no-brainers. They've been well-publicised in the mainstream for years—and are obvious as being detrimental to the environment. However, the effect of animal agriculture on the environment has historically been a hidden entity in the mainstream.

Now, it's slowly becoming more mainstream and is understood to be one of the leading contributors to various pollution statistics worldwide. Many people are starting to recognise that to nip this in the bud, they need to take action. So, a plant-based diet is often depicted as a "futuristic" diet. For the good of your children, children's children, children's children's children, etc.

By sticking to this diet, you won't get a medal, but you may get a great sense of self-satisfaction knowing that every day, your decisions are going to a natural cause. The more you look into it, the more you'll realise what I mean.

The Vegan Calculator website estimates that by adopting a plant-based diet for just one day, you will save: 1,100 gallons of water, 40 lbs of grain, 30 sq. feet of forest, 20 lbs of co2, and one animal life. **thevegancalculator.com**

When I looked back at this a year down the line, it really made me see the benefits on animals and the environment, which will continue compounding as I stick to the diet and talk to others about it. Every year, you will save: 396,000 gallons of water, 14,400 lbs of grain, 10,800 sq. feet of forest, 7,200 lbs of co2, and 365 animal lives.

"Plants feel pain"

There are four different topics that can bring light to this misconception:

The definition of sentience.
The nervous system.
The definition of pain.
The natural response to pain.

Do plants have the ability to perceive or feel things? In other words, are they sentient beings like humans and animals?

Charles Darwin is thought to have studied plants meticulously for decades. He was one of the first scientists to recognise that plants move and respond to sensation. They are inclined to grow towards sources of water and light, which they need to survive. Basically, proving that they are sentient. It's thought that plants face many of the same problems as animals, though they differ significantly in their approach. Similar to animals, plants have to find energy, reproduce, and stave off predators too!

If this is the case, and plants are indeed able to perceive or feel things, then why has plant sentience been ignored for so long? Essentially, it's because the majority of people would most likely argue that plants aren't sentient at all. This makes it easier to completely ignore plant sentience. The other reason is because humans simply can't relate to plants given how different they are to humans and animals. It's almost impossible to imagine what your life would be like if you were a plant, isn't it!?

So, do plants have a nervous system? One study suggested that plants can transmit information from leaf to leaf in a very similar way to the human nervous system. They can supposedly even think and remember.

The study explained that the big mistake people make is speaking as if plants "know" what they're doing. Researchers rather describe it as a plant "senses and responds". So, plants don't have a nervous system as we know it, but they do have something else.

Do plants feel pain? Researchers suggest not trying to compare humans and animals to plants if looking to get to the bottom of this. However, when we think of pain and natural responses to it, we can only relate to how humans or animals would react. When it comes to plants, we have to assume that they would react similarly, but in their own way. To say that plants feel pain suggests that plants suffer, which means they are capable of emotional stress. Naturally, we think of what emotional stress is like for humans and animals. Ultimately, we end up comparing and looking out for similar activity to prove whether plants feel pain or not. So it's quite difficult to come to a conclusion for this particular question.

You'll come across this "plants feel pain" thing fairly often in the mainstream, as people look to have banter with, or be cynical about, vegans. Whether or not you care about plants feeling pain, what's important is whether you understand the agenda behind the misconception. Where people are pretty much insinuating that if you eat plants instead of animals because you don't want to inflict pain and suffering, then you may still be inflicting pain and suffering to plants. In which case, they see it as though you might as well eat animals.

Looking at animals differently than before

One day, I was at a farm and the farmer had chickens. They weren't caged, so I guess you could call them free range. There was around ten. I stood by the enclosure and looked at the chickens. They were looking at me. It was a weird moment. The chickens probably thought I was a bit weird for staring at them! I'm not too proud to admit that I loved the taste of meat. But seeing the chickens all chickeny like that made me feel sick. You can probably tell, I didn't grow up on a farm!

Prior to that experience, I had never registered the correlation between a living, clucking chicken with eyes that look right into yours, and my mum's chicken fajitas for example. This is of course just the tip of the iceberg when you think of how ever-present chicken is across mainstream food.

I had to wonder, why hadn't I registered this before? I'd felt a sense of "enlightenment" since I last saw a chicken, and it was the first time I'd seen a regularly-eaten animal in the flesh since beginning my transition to a plant-based diet. One that I used to eat my fair share of!

It's just so different seeing an animal you used to eat alive in the flesh, with moving eyes, lots of hair, and a weird, red flappy ballbag for a neck—not just as shiny meat in a packet.

"Humans are top of the food chain"

In the food chain, ecologists rank species by their diets using a metric called the trophic level:

- Plants, which produce their own food, are given a rank of 1.
- Herbivores, which eat only plants, are ranked 2.
- The fiercest of carnivores, such as killer whales, rank at 5.5.

In 2013, the average global human trophic level (HTL) was 2.21. This puts the human diet on par with pigs and anchovies. 2.5 would mean that the human diet is split evenly between plants and herbivores (such as cows). A diet of 2.21 means that humans still generally eat far more plants than meat.

It's thought that the HTL number for humans would be even lower, however in recent times, poorer countries such as China and India have become wealthier, so have chosen to eat more meat, which has increased the global HTL. Africa and Southeast Asia have relatively low HTLs, and the U.S. and Western Europe have relatively high HTLs. The highest HTLs go to Mongolia, Sweden, and Finland, where diets are mostly fish- and meat-based. Vegetables in these countries are generally considered an afterthought.

Going by tropic levels, you could say that humans aren't top of the food chain. That said, I believe that they are, and you may feel this way too. Reason being, humans have ways of taming animals and fish. Big, small, aggressive, evasive, and so on. When I say "taming", it isn't just our ability to domesticate an animal and change its behaviour, like dogs or cats. Or even exotic animals such as lions, tigers, bears, and elephants in circuses. Or sharks, crocodiles, and killer whales in aquariums. But also in other means of taming: making something less powerful and easier to control.

By contrast, animals don't seem to coerce other animals or humans in the same way as humans do to them. Especially animals higher up the food chain. Instead, animals have a more direct approach to "taming", mostly via brute force and primal instinct. This is often based on what they must do to achieve certain credentials in their environment, such as status and territory.

If you look at the more dominant members of a species in the animal kingdom, they are usually the biggest, strongest, and most aggressive of their age group. These more dominant members ones then compete against each other for dominance of their troop. Humans, on the other hand, tend to want to dominate all species. Not just their own. You could say that this isn't a good thing, given the rapid decline of other species.

It's true that extinction is a natural phenomenon, and more than 90% of all organisms that have ever lived on Earth are now extinct. However, history tells us that extinction should occur at a natural background rate of around 1-5 species per year. Scientists estimate that we're now losing species at 1,000 to 10,000 times the background rate, with dozens going extinct every day. At this rate, a possible 30-50% of all species will be heading towards extinction by mid-century.

With this is mind, just because we've made our way to the top of the food chain by taming animals higher up the tropic food chain than us, should we be taking advantage of this and eating them? I'll leave that for you to decide.

Eating A LOT more fruit than ever before

I didn't realise how much fruit I was eating a day until one of my clients asked me. During the conversation, I tried to work it out as we spoke and came to the conclusion that it was around 10 pieces a day. Plus drinking a glass of fruit juice (not from concentrate). Only a few months before, I'd been eating a very conservative few pieces a day, mostly around training and exercise, and opting for lower G.I fruits. This had escalated somewhat!

I was mostly consuming bananas, apples, oranges, kiwis, raspberries, strawberries, blackberries, and blueberries. Not just on their own, but as different combinations mixed with oats and nut butters. As many as possible basically!

I intentionally ate more fruits than I drank, as juicing often removes the fibre and other nutrients such as vitamin C. It's also known to elevate blood sugar levels more rapidly than whole fruit, potentially making you hungry sooner.

With my new-found love of fruit, my first instinct was that I'd been depriving myself. Not just of flavour, but also of nutrients. My concentration, focus, and energy levels were on a different scale than ever before. I was wondering, why hadn't I ever aimed to consume more than 5 a day before? Or why hadn't I made a banging fruit cocktail to snack on between clients? Oh yeah...carbs!

Fruit = sugar. Sugar makes you fat. Although the carb thing was still in the back of my mind, the reality was I had actually lost weight again. Not much. But a couple of kg. I realised I was near my leanest ever and had lower body fat—without even trying. Again, I hadn't been aware of living in a calorie deficit. The interesting thing was that I had more energy than ever before by eating less. Was this due to the micronutrients? Yes, but also a big thanks to eating more carbs.

Reducing my overall fat intake was responsible for my calorie deficit, as fat is much higher in calories than carbs. There's 9kcal per 1g of fat to 4kcal to 1g of carbs. I thought I'd been piling on the calories through the increased fruit consumption. But actually, fruit isn't that high in calories. For example, two apples is only 100kcal. Fruit also contains a lot of fibre, which fills you up and may prevent binging. Unlike biscuits and sweets, which contain next to no fibre, so you're still hungry and end up eating the whole packet.

After noticing my calorie deficit through weight loss and an app called Cronometer (which I was now using in place of MyFitnessPal), I saw where the rest of my micronutrients could be coming from. I recommend this app if you want to see your micronutrient intake in greater detail - **cronometer.com**

However, these lacking micronutrients (vitamin B6, vitamin B12, vitamin D, iron, some amino acids, and omega 3 and 6 fatty acids) couldn't be accounted for in my diet by eating more fruit, as they didn't contain them. All the notorious mainstream vegan deficiencies.

No biggy! It was all relatively new to me, I had basically got a little too happy with fruit and wasn't making ends meet elsewhere in the day. Thankfully, I could nip it in the bud early. So, I began to research ways to make up for these missing nutrients elsewhere and cut back on the fruit intake. The good news was I wouldn't have to eat less overall, but actually eat more to reach my body composition and micronutrient goals. Fine by me!

"5 a day is all you need"

The 5 A Day campaign is based on advice from the World Health Organisation. They recommend eating a minimum of 400g of fruit and vegetables a day to lower the risk of serious health problems, such as heart disease, stroke, and some cancers. The number 5 came from evidence that shows there are significant health benefits in getting at least five 80g portions of fruit and vegetables every day. A single 80g portion is along the lines of 1 small banana, 1 apple, 1 pear, or another similar sized fruit; 2 plums, 2 satsumas, 2 kiwis, or another similar sized fruit, etc.

On a plant-based diet, you may expect to consume more fruit and vegetables than the average person, because your other choices are limited. But is 5 portions a day enough? Are there any health benefits in eating more than 5 portions per day? Would it be even better if you consumed 5 portions of fruit and 5 portions of vegetables a day?

First of all, some people may not be getting 5 a day. The average reported in the UK is more like 4 a day. Getting some fruit and vegetables is better than getting none, surely? The good news is, a study found that even a daily intake of 200g (or two and a half standard 80g portions) is associated with the following risk reductions: 16% for heart disease, 18% for stroke, 13% for cardiovascular disease, 4% for cancer, and 15% in premature deaths.

Secondly, these campaigns differ from country to country. In Australia, official health advice encourages people to eat 2 helpings of fruit and 5 portions of vegetables a day. This may be because fresh vegetables are found to have the strongest protective effect, followed by salad, then fruit. Eating salad is a super convenient way to get multiple fruits and veggies in one hit.

So, what about more than the recommended 5 a day? Eating up to 800g of fruit and vegetables a day (the equivalent of 10 portions) was associated with the following risk reductions: 24% for heart disease, 33% for stroke, 28% for cardiovascular disease, 13% for cancer overall, and 31% in premature deaths. Unlike the Australian study, UK researchers reported no difference between the protective effects of cooked vs. raw fruit and vegetables.

The best at preventing heart disease and stroke are apples, pears, citrus fruits, salads, green leafy vegetables such as spinach and lettuce, and cruciferous vegetables such as broccoli, cabbage, and cauliflower. The best at reducing the risk of cancer are green vegetables such as green beans, yellow and orange vegetables such as peppers and carrots, and cruciferous vegetables such as broccoli.

It all sounds great, doesn't it!? But where do you stop with the fruit intake? Ultimately, your limit is when you've hit your caloric, macro, and micronutrient targets for your goals every day. Then, you can say that you've eaten enough to reach your goals. This will differ from person to person.

Understandably the sugar thing may also come into it, as some people are put off by the idea of consuming more sugar, albeit in the form of fruit. In this case, the total amount you consume to reach your daily targets is a personal preference based on your goals. You can use MyFitnessPal or Chronometer to help with this as it will outline recommended daily allowances, or you can talk to a Nutritionist or Personal Trainer with qualifications in nutrition to tailor this to you.

Getting used to all the new fibre

There are two types of fibre, and both play a different role in the body

- Soluble fibre: This type dissolves in water to form a gel-like material in the gut. It can help to slow digestion, and lower blood cholesterol and blood sugar levels. This type is typically related to brown or wholegrain foods, though there are a variety of sources to soluble fibre. So, people generally think of this as being found in grains.

- Insoluble fibre: This type promotes the movement of material through the digestive system. It can speed up digestion, and help with constipation and regular bowel movements. Similar to soluble fibre, there are many sources, but it's mostly known to be found in fruit, seeds, and nuts.

Most plant-based foods contain both types of fibre, and it's important to get a variety of both. Some foods have a more dominant type than the other, while other foods have very similar amounts of both types.

We already looked at how fibre makes you go to the toilet more. The other thing it potentially causes is bloating. Bloating is a generic term for any type of pressure caused by gas or air in your stomach or chest. It often leads to burping or flatulence, but it may also cause chest pains, abdominal pains, pressure, constipation, and more.

Personally, bloating was relatively new territory since making the transition. Probably because I consumed barely any fibre before! But naturally, it gave me a few concerns about keeping up the diet. Sometimes, increasing my water intake made it worse. Other times, I couldn't even eat because it was so uncomfortable. I tried a few techniques to alleviate it, such as:

- Increasing my exercise levels to increase my demand for calories.
- Intermittent fasting—a pattern of eating that involves fasting and eating over set periods of time.
- Reducing my caffeine intake and sometimes avoiding caffeine altogether.
- Drinking boiled warm water instead of tap water.
- Reducing my bread intake.
- Chewing my food for longer.

The great thing is that they all helped to an extent. But the thing that always worked was not eating big meal after big meal. Something I was guilty of before, as I had been reckless with the quantities of food meal after meal. It turned out that eating less in one sitting was the most effective technique. For me, this was around a quarter less. If you ever feel bloated, I'd recommend going through the points above and also paying attention to your portion sizes.

"All vegans eat is fruit and vegetables"

Vegans generally eat any food as long as it's plant-based. As we know, this includes more food types than just fruits and vegetables. Nuts, seeds, beans, legumes, and grains are all plant-based foods too.

While there is no set-in-stone vegan diet, there are different "types" if you will, and this is probably where the misconception comes from. All vegans are different, with individual diets, but some people compartmentalise the diet into more specifics than the "general vegan" approach.

This is usually done to manufacture a popular diet or lifestyle in the mainstream. Just like you see with the conventional Western diet. For example, the Atkins diet, the 5-2 diet, and the Paleo diet. These are all spin-offs or versions of society's most popular diet. Some followers of the Paleo diet refer to themselves as "a Paleo", and there are certain rules to abide by.

So, some people class their diet as a certain type of diet, and some vegans class themselves as a certain type of vegan. The thing to take on board is that all types of vegan diet indicate the main agenda behind the vegan diet and fall into the vegan category by definition: a way of living that seeks to exclude, as far as is possible and practicable, all forms of exploitation of, and cruelty to, animals for food, clothing, or any other purpose.

There are many examples, but the most popular vegan spin-off versions are:

Junk food vegans:

This type tends to be vegans for ethical rather than health reasons. Any food is fair game as long as it doesn't include animal products. As it may also include plant-based foods, it may not all be junk food, but there is often a lack of structure in their nutrition. The diet generally doesn't tie into performance or body composition related goals. Because of this, this type of vegan is seen to be unhealthy. This can cause confusion in the mainstream about the health benefits of a plant-based diet.

Some people go through the junk food phase when first transitioning to a plant-based diet. Then they find out that just being vegan-friendly doesn't make something healthy! This diet isn't massively a bad thing in the short term. Until you've upped your knowledge on plant-based nutrition, it gives you peace of mind while you adjust. Just don't get too comfortable here!

HCLF (high-carb, low-fat):

This involves getting around 80% of the total daily calories from carbs, up to 10% from protein, and up to 10% from fats. This diet has been linked to more athletic people, specifically endurance athletes. Their physiques tend to be very lean and slim, confusing the "carbs make you fat" belief even more!

The guidelines for this diet are that the vast majority of total daily calories come from carbs, not fat or protein. As such, fruit and vegetables are usually the mainstay, along with some grains such as rice. There are no boundaries on whether carbs come from sugar or not.

The big difference between this diet and a traditional raw food diet is the emphasis on keeping fat content low. This means avoiding disproportionate quantities of nuts, seeds, avocados, and oils for example, relevant to the total daily calorie intake.

Whole foods/plant-based:

This type is often regarded as the most health-conscious. They tend to stick to unprocessed foods, preferably organic, and try to avoid anything that comes in a packet, unless it's got the right kind of goods inside of course. They often avoid common irritants such as GMO, oil, refined sugar, and other chemicals. Some also attempt to avoid irritants such as gluten and soy. This type tends to cook and prepare food from scratch at home and take it out with them.

I've met many people who classify themselves as plant-based or on a whole food diet to avoid the stigma of the vegan diet. As you may have guessed, I try to stick to this style wherever possible. Fortunately, I quite enjoy healthy food, well the benefits of it more so than the taste anyway! That said, not everyone does, and some aspects of this type won't appeal to everyone.

Raw vegans:

Raw vegans eat much or all of their food raw, or heated/dehydrated at very low temperatures. Basically, they don't cook very often! This means they will generally eat fruit, salad, raw vegetables, nuts, seeds, and nut butters. Depending on their level of rawness, dehydrated snacks such as flax crackers and rice cakes could also be on the menu. Often, people who follow this diet switch between different levels of rawness at various stages of their lives. There are also 100% all-in raw vegans, who have been for some time.

Whichever type of vegan diet, the general consensus is increased consumption of fruit and veg. Sometimes, you'll have no other choice when looking for foods in the mainstream. On the flip side, sometimes you'll have no other choice but to eat junk if those choices aren't available!

Supplements

Despite tracking my micronutrients through Cronometer and keeping my macronutrients close to my goals, the mainstream hysteria about nutrient deficiency in the vegan diet still had me buying into the idea that I could be doing better. The keyword being "buying", as I was more prepared to buy a supplement than do further research into foods that could give me an edge.

The supplements that turned my head to begin with were vegan-friendly protein powders. That "P word" again! I weighed up the options, their benefits, and the prices. From that, I went with hemp protein.

At first, I took it as recommended: daily and when I needed protein, like after training. The only differences were being more bloated, farting more, and going to the toilet more! So, I took it every other day instead. The same thing happened. It was unnecessary and self-inflicted. So, I switched to every few days. The same thing. Then only occasionally in smoothies. Same again.

I'm not just hating on hemp protein—as soy, brown rice, and pea protein all had the same effect on me. It's not just vegan-friendly protein powders either. Back in the day, whey protein did the same to me, only ten times worse!

After that, I experimented with green powders to provide essential nutrients, including vitamins, minerals, and amino acids that don't appear so conveniently in my diet. At least not all in one hit. These supplements include a combination of spirulina, wheatgrass, chlorella, kale, broccoli, beetroot, and alfalfa powder. I still have these once or twice a week, as I got past the initial digestive symptoms.

I dabble in energy gels and electrolyte tablets for endurance training, and enjoy the benefits, especially on long runs. Strangely, vegan-friendly protein bars don't seem to affect me like the powders do. If I'm doing more resistance training or training more frequently, I'll crack open a tub of protein powder and/or take vegan-friendly amino acids as my body will require more protein. It's just super convenient during busier times and the digestive issues don't seem to be as common if I genuinely create a demand for it. The protein I go for is usually a blend of vegan protein sources as I have no specific preference at the time of writing this.

Other supplements I'll dabble in include vitamin B12, vitamin

D3 (the sunshine vitamin—not much of that in London!) and omega-3s (EPA and DHA). In theory, I don't get much of these elsewhere in my diet and may potentially struggle to make ends meet, so I take them for peace of mind. I'll also take an effervescent high-strength multivitamin from time to time if my work load is high and sleep quality not as good.

For me, the best results I have ever got (performance, mood, and digestion related) always come from eating better. It goes back to staying on top of your nutrition, managing what you're eating at home and out, and considering your goals. Food prep plays a big part in this. Within this, supplements may come in handy from time to time, but they shouldn't be the foundation.

"Vegans need to supplement with vitamin B12"

Getting enough B12 is important, as the largest and most complex vitamin currently known. B12 is required for proper red blood cell formation, neurological function, and DNA synthesis. A deficiency, albeit only slight, is thought to lead to anaemia, fatigue, and depression. Long-term deficiency may cause permanent damage to the brain and central nervous system.

Symptoms can take five years or more to develop in adults, though some people experience problems within a year. A very small number of individuals avoid clinical deficiency symptoms for 20 years or more.

Vitamin B12 can only be manufactured by bacteria and can only be found naturally in animal products, including fish, meat, poultry, eggs, milk, and milk products. As such, vegans are thought to be at greater risk of developing a B12 deficiency. That said, synthetic forms are widely available and added to many foods that vegans can eat. So, it's thought that most vegans consume enough B12 to avoid a clinical deficiency. However, two subgroups of vegans are at particular risk: long-term vegans who avoid common fortified foods (such as raw vegans) and breastfed infants of vegan mothers whose intake of B12 is low.

Simply put, if you're not eating enough calories, macronutrients, and/or micronutrients such as vitamin B12 or iron, you will develop fatigue at some point. The current RDA of vitamin B12 for adults (14+) is 2.4mcg. This is lower for younger individuals and higher for pregnant women. The most potent sources of B12 include: sea lion liver, molluscs, abalone, beef liver, lamb liver, veal liver, walrus liver, seal liver, veal, and lamb kidneys. So not the most popular of foods then!

Synthetic forms are found in supplements. They can also be found in fortified foods. Fortified mean that extra nutrients have been added. The original purpose of fortifying food was to decrease nutrient deficiencies. For example, child and pregnant women may need more of certain nutrient than others. Pretty much any micronutrient can be fortified to suit these requirements.

Fortified foods vary, so it's important to read the product label to see which added nutrients they contain, and how much. Fortified foods include cereal, milk, tofu, nutritional yeast, and yeast spread. You may find that a fortified cereal provides 100% RDA of vitamin B12 per serving. If it has less, then you know how much more you need to consume to get your RDA.

If the product says it "may contain B12", then it may not! This goes for food such as spirulina, because any bacteria removed in the manufacturing process effectively removes the B12—unless it is fortified.

So, do you need to take a B12 supplement in addition to eating fortified foods? Vegan or not, it's recommend that anyone who doesn't consume adequate B12 from fortified foods or animal products should take a supplement. However, supplements aren't thought to be as well-absorbed as fortified foods, so the preference is to consume it from food before resorting to supplements. I take both for good measure.

Wishing I had done this sooner

Not long after my transition to the final stage, I started running to prepare for an upcoming obstacle course race I'd entered with a few clients. I couldn't believe how good long-distance running felt considering how little I had run in the past. I'd done a couple of similar events before and trained a fair few clients for these events, but this time, I was hitting long-distance PBs out of nowhere and felt like I had been running for years.

The most notable increases in my physical performance came from endurance sports such as running and indoor cycling. These sports are very much associated with mental, as well as physical endurance. This is why so many people don't enjoy them! Endurance is defined as: The ability to endure an unpleasant or difficult process or situation without giving way.

My mental endurance since adopting a plant-based diet wasn't exclusively in sport. It was also benefiting me at the desk, and in my other work duties. I could concentrate for longer periods and work much more efficiently, with real intent. I delivered higher standards in each and every PT session, because I felt fitter and more switched on from start to finish.

Being optimistic most of the time, I tried my best to not become resentful that I hadn't done this sooner. I started thinking, do you blame yourself? Do you blame the media? Do you blame the system? Do you blame evolution? Sounds bizarre, I know. I just didn't know where to turn! After a little deliberation, the realisation struck: it was time to feel fortunate that I had found this diet, instead of resentful that it taken so long to clock on.

"Vegans are in denial about their health and are too stubborn to change"

My quest to understand this misconception led me to an interesting podcast. A guest on the podcast suggested that a plant-based diet was only healthy in the short term, and in the long term, it meant a higher chance of getting ill.

His theory was: because plant-based foods are so high in micronutrients and carbs, your body doesn't realise how much it's getting in terms of calories and protein. As such, it acts as a smokescreen to what your body really needs. Because the diet is new, you feel good and energised. But in the long term, you get ill because you're not eating enough or getting enough protein (particularly animal), so you feel weak. There were also lots of references to the healthy fat in fish as being essential for omega-3 conversion.

His overall point was: even if vegans identify they're better on a non-vegan diet, they will be in denial and too stubborn to change. Like they become reckless with their own health. The validity of his insights was supposedly research and experience. Apparently, he was a vegan once upon a time, before realising his diet was making him ill. He played devil's advocate by saying that not all vegan diets are bad, and some people such as athletes pull it off well, but for it to work, you have to get every detail spot on. In that, he undermined his own argument that vegan diets are generally bad.

Of course, I had to look further into this. A U.S. study of 11,399 adults found that 37% of former vegetarians and vegans would go back to their diet. If it was that bad for them, why would they want to try it again? And why couldn't they sustain it the first time? The main cause for not sustaining it was finding it difficult to be "pure" with their diet (43%), while 29% said they experienced specific health-related symptoms during their diet. Again, this is likely down to the individual's nutritional choices. In both cases, this could probably be resolved through proper education and preparation.

I couldn't speak much from experience, as I'd only been on the plant-based diet for about six months or so. But I wondered how long it would take to reach the stubborn stage of no return! Then I thought, I'm eating to my goals: calories, protein, carbs, and fat all in check, and eating more micronutrients than ever before. Cronometer shows I'm getting omega-3 in too. I'm the fittest ever, both mentally and physically. I'm doing the best ever in my business. I'm the happiest and most positive I've ever been. So what am I missing out on from my diet before? Isn't the goal of nutrition to feel the way I feel now?

Then I realised the guy in the podcast wasn't talking about vegans at all. He was talking about himself. He was just using the vegan thing to explain where he went wrong in his nutritional decisions. He had buyer's remorse and clearly wasn't eating to his goals.

I do empathise with him, because he didn't get his plant-based diet right for him. And not everyone will—not everyone who reads this will either. But who do you blame for that, the diet or the individual? Deep down, many people will only blame themselves if they're being completely honest.

First BBQ as a vegan

A friend invited me to a BBQ at his house with some of our friends, my first since the meat days! I was really looking forward to seeing them. But I was worried that given the "meaty" environment, my different food choices would be highlighted, and most or all of my friends just wouldn't "get it".

Beforehand, I decided there was no need to explain myself. Likewise, I certainly didn't want to turn up to a BBQ where everyone was eating meat and shout my head off that you shouldn't eat meat, because it's bad for you, the environment, and the animals that have to suffer horrendously. So, I stayed quiet about my change in diet and mingled as normal.

They only picked up on it when it came to eating time and I had something different, when they had meat, cheese, quiche, pork pies, scotch eggs, etc. Of course, some of the gang were inquisitive. Individually, no one asked much about it. But as a group, a few tried to engage while we were eating. If asked, I kept it confidently vague, especially in my reasoning. No more detail than: "Yeah I've been doing it for a while" and "Yeah, it feels great."

The fact that I brought my own food really helped. It appeared that I came prepared and no one had to make a fuss to suit my nutritional requirements. This differentiated me from the "typical vegan" they imagined, who would kick up a fuss and be awkward.

I thought about the rule of reciprocity, which in social psychology is defined as: a social rule that says people should repay, in kind, what another person has provided for them. People will give back (reciprocate) the kind of treatment they have received from another.

A study said the average person spends around £35 on food and drink for a BBQ. So, I bought a generous serving of homemade salad for everyone as a gesture that we're still a group regardless of me eating differently. I ended up spending £20, because there's only so much salad you can bring to a BBQ!

In this instance, it showed an unselfishness, caring attitude. Bringing food—even though you're probably not going to be eating the same food as everyone else—shows this attitude. It may come as a pleasant surprise to some people, who might have expected that as a vegan, you won't be looking out for those who eat meat.

"Vegan food prep is expensive"

What you deem to be expensive is dependent on your income and how highly you value your health. Whichever way you look at it, this misconception is based on individual circumstances. Like do you have the disposable income to spend on certain food?

One study found that healthy food (fruit and veg) costs three times as much as junk food (high in calories, fat, and sugar). This was based on the standard way of assessing food poverty: measuring calories, not vitamin and mineral content.

However, healthy food tends to have fewer calories per gram (lower energy density) than junk foods, so this measure may not provide a realistic comparison. For example, you would need to eat around 30 cucumbers to gain 1,000 calories compared to one 200g packet of ginger nut biscuits. This seems to be a good thing if you want to lose weight because eating 30 cucumbers is difficult whereas eating a packet of biscuits would be easy! But it could also be seen as a bad thing if you need to eat sufficient calories from healthy foods because it will cost more.

- Between 2002–2012, 94 healthy foods increased in price more rapidly than less healthy foods (around £7.49 vs. £2.50 for 1,000kcal of each).
- The comparative price was always highest for fruit and veg, lowest for starchy foods (bread, rice, potatoes, and pasta), and second lowest for those high in fat and/or sugar.
- The price of meat increased by 26% between 2007-2016, and fish saw an increase in price of 31%.
- The price of starchy foods stayed roughly the same over 10 years, while the other groups increased in price.

A 2015 UK research study found that workers could save £1300 a year if they made sandwiches for work at home, rather than buying them from a shop. As such, if you compare the price of buying food on the go meal to meal vs. buying food in bulk and prepping it in advance, the latter is easily the least expensive, even when factoring in that healthy food may be more expensive. From personal experience, I've seen that this is true, as buying food in bulk is cheaper than buying as you go. If you prep at home, you can get your daily food spend down to just a few pounds.

So, you can save money by prepping your food in advance. However, we have to face facts that overall, healthy food may be more expensive. That said, if you can afford to make healthier choices, then you should. And by cutting out meat and animal products, you should have more money to spend on healthy food.

Taking criticism and compliments at the same time

As you get more experience and learn how to best conduct yourself around other people when it comes to your diet, you may be surprised at the marmite effect you create. There are times when you wonder whether someone is being nice or a dick. And you may question whether people have ulterior motives with their conversation, like they're secretly trying to mug you off.

It's thought that communication in person is only 7% verbal and 93% non-verbal. The non-verbal component is made up of 55% body language and 38% tone of voice. With this in mind, I really dialled in on my mannerisms. I knew I'd been acting pretty cool about the diet, because people had told me so. That said, a few people were still out to debunk me and my diet.

The marmite effect kicked in around this time. I had made lots of new friends and built great relationships with people—just as much as I'd lost with others. The most significant change came from people who were on the fence about me anyway. People who weren't really my friends. Whether this was down to change in diet or change in aura because of the diet, I couldn't tell you!

Either way, I loved this because it made everything clearer. It showed me who was and wasn't my real friend, and really helped me crack on with the other things in life. I learned very quickly not to take criticism on my diet to heart, and not let the compliments go to my head!

"Vegans are weak"

To evaluate this misconception, we first need to define "weak". It could be defined in a few different ways. If weak means the opposite of strong, then we need to define what exactly is considered to be strength. Does it mean the ability to pick up heavy stuff, i.e. physical strength? Or the ability to keep going through tough times, i.e. mental strength?

If weak means "weakness", then we need to identify what exactly weakness is considered to be. Does it mean a guilty pleasure that you can't resist, like chocolate? Or does it mean an injury, like an old back strain that comes back if you're not careful?

When people attempt to say that vegans are weak, it basically means "vegans are inferior to normal people". It's a comparison. Much of the time, this ties back into the assumption that a plant-based diet means no protein, or not the right type of protein, or you're going to get skinny, or lose muscle.

Many people only see it as big muscles = strong. Or lifting heavy weights = strength. They don't identify the other possible definitions. Of course, big muscles = strong and lifting heavy weights = strength can be right, because both can represent strength. But it strength can also mean so much more.

Personally, I define many things as being strength, not just what meets the eye like big muscles and lifting heavy weights. Determination and intelligence are also strength. I also define many things as being weakness, not just what meets the eye like being skinny or not lifting heavy weights. Giving up on your goals easily and being ignorant towards personal development could be an example of weakness.

There are many athletes competing at the highest level of their sport who are on a fully plant-based diet. From strength- and endurance-based sports such as Olympic weightlifting and ultra-marathon running to team sports such as football, and competitive sports such as tennis and mixed martial arts. Some have gone public about their diet, and others haven't. There are also everyday heroes (not in the public eye) who eat a plant-based diet and are smashing life to their own standards.

To say that vegans are weak based on appearance and physical performance in comparison to non-vegans isn't useful. Comparisons are useless without identifying exactly what the point of comparison is. Having done this, you may realise that it doesn't come down to vegan vs. non-vegan and is more often related to the individual, their commitment, and their skillset.

Is it okay to laugh at vegan parodies?

Vegan parodies are basically piss-takes! Some of them are ridiculous internet things created by trolls, which you may even laugh at. However, sometimes you might shake your head, as these people really don't get what it's all about.

Some of it can be seen as quite offensive. For a while, I wasn't sure how to react. This is the kind of stuff circulating on social media:

Hashtags:
#StopVegans: Where vegans are eating all the plants and destroying Earth.
#AntiVegan: Where people post pictures of meat.
#Vegan: Where people post pictures of meat.

Parody videos:
For example, "If meat eaters acted like vegans", which displays a generalisation of a vegan based on mainstream beliefs. And "Vegan of 30 years eats meat for the first time", which displays a fake vegan eating meat and crying tears of joy.

Memes:

For example, a picture of a human mouth, pointing out the canines, or "vegetarian is ancient tribal slang for the village idiot who couldn't catch its prey", as we covered earlier. Memes have eye-catching writing or a photo to get your attention—but don't be gullible enough to believe everything you read!

Online comments:

Someone on my Facebook feed posted "vegans are the worst" on a vegan parody video that went viral. Another comment was: "my food eats your food". The comments on YouTube videos are usually the most savage!

Without sounding like I'm pulling out the "vegan card", unfair discrimination against vegans does exist. I've experienced some shockingly weird discrimination and ridicule. But because people don't see it as illegal discrimination and it's seen as funny by the mainstream, then it will keep happening.

In all honesty, you have to be fairly thick-skinned on a plant-based diet, because there are no societal boundaries if someone takes the piss out of you. Who's going to stop them? Imagine calling the police and telling them you want to make a complaint because someone has called you a "vegan" and questioned your motives for eating plant-based food. The police would laugh their heads off! Bottom line is, nobody will take your complaint seriously, so you've got to deal with it in your own way.

Some of my friends and family regularly tag me in vegan parodies because they think it's funny and think I'll see the funny side. Truth be told, I don't even watch them as they're often a million miles away from the truth and are attention-seeking. So, I can't be bothered. That's basically how I deal with vegan parodies—I don't give them time of day!

As plant-based diets become better understood by the majority, you'll likely still see these parodies, but on a lesser scale. I believe we'll definitely see less engagement within them. Partly because people will have seen it all before, but also because more people will connect with the benefits of the diet. And because some of the misconceptions will be quashed in the mainstream. Whether you laugh at them or not is your choice!

"Vegans care more about animals than they do humans"

I think you'll agree that humans are bastards sometimes and can put you off other people. But you don't have to be a vegan to hate people. If anything, chances are that if you're vegan, you'll have more compassion in general, because if you care about animals, why wouldn't you care about humans? It just shows you're not afraid of the love, man!

From my own experience of going from meat eater to vegan, I believe that non-vegans often see meat, whereas vegans see animals. I think this is where the mainstay of "vegans care about animals more" comes from, because vegans give off a different vibe to the majority on the subject. Vegans are often more aware of elements surrounding speciesism and animal equality, because they've researched it, and this breeds further differentiation in society.

Besides this, stigmatism comes from protests and charities. When vegans are protesting for animal rights, some people see it as unnecessary or less important in the grand scheme of things, when there are wars going on around the world, terrorism on the streets, political scandals, and many other life-altering events that directly impact a human's quality of life.

Charities can be portrayed in the same context, because supporting animal rights isn't such a priority to some people compared to charities that support human welfare. However, supporting animal charities doesn't mean you like animals more than people. Maybe supporters of animal charities just want to help. Plus, who's to say they don't also support human-focused charities too?

Whichever way you look at it, whether someone cares more about animals than humans is a personal preference. You don't have to be a vegan to prefer animals or dislike humans. And you don't have to prefer animals to be a vegan.

I'm living proof of this. It never even crosses my mind whether I prefer animals or humans. I like both. I care enough about humans to help them transition to a plant-based diet if they want to. And I care enough about animals not to eat them!

Going on holiday

Picture this: Summer. Stag do. Ibiza. 20 friends. All who love to partaaay. You the vegan. And you don't even drink. How'd do you reckon that went?

To be certain of vegan-friendly snacks for the holiday, I checked out the local mini-supermarket when we arrived in the early hours. The best and most suitable snacks were some nice-looking fruit, unsalted varieties of nuts, bottled water, juices not from concentrate, freshly-made bread, and hummus. This is going to be a doddle, I thought to myself. Sorted.

But what about eating out? In all honesty, I really fucking struggled with it. My basic GCSE German wasn't going to help here! There were a few not-so-successful orders at your typical cafe/grill restaurants, where meat or cheese rocked up with my supposed "vegan-friendly" meal. After that, along with a health-conscious friend, we sloped off from the group to find a healthier place to eat. We picked a funky place that had a vegetarian option and served smoothies.

I ordered what seemed like the least-complicated meal on the menu and that would suit my nutritional requirements: wilted spinach, avocado, mushrooms, tomatoes, fresh granary bread, and eggs. Sounds pretty suitable right, minus the eggs? In theory, all that needed to happen was: take the eggs out.

Having done my best with the server, they seemed to understand "vegan-friendly" (though so had all the other places that had fucked up the order) and agreed to take the eggs out. I tried to get more of something else to replace it, but they stressed they don't do that. No dramas. We ate our meal. It was 6/10. The smoothie was a 9. At least it was all vegan-friendly.

But when the bill came, something didn't add up. Upon closer inspection, they had added extra on my meal. Only a few euros, but enough to be noticed. I politely called for the server and bless her, she had to explain that it's one of the restaurants policies to charge extra if anything is to taken out of the meal. She seemed embarrassed, but authoritative. I had to laugh (fake laugh). You get less, but you pay more. Seems reasonable. I paid anyway.

After that, my confidence in keeping things vegan-friendly had taken a massive knock. I didn't know where to turn for a hot meal. I could have lived off the snacks in the mini-supermarket, but it was a holiday, and I wanted to have food cooked for me for a change. So, I thought, better the devil you know! There was a Subway nearby, and plenty around. I needed consistency, no stress, and to just get what I'd asked for. It had reached the point I just wanted a warm sandwich. Wasn't exactly asking for much, was I?

One of the options that seemed vegan-friendly was a "veggie patty", a veggie burger type thing. It was that or "veggie delight", which was literally nothing but bread and salad. I assumed the veggie patty was just vegetables and therefore vegan-friendly because of its name, and thought that by dodging the cheese and creamy sauce, the meal would be suitable.

Thanks to the veggie patty discovery, I visited Subway on a daily basis, getting a footlong with all the salad, hot chilli sauce, no cheese, and no dodgy sauce that had animal products in it. I began to see Subway like an oasis in the desert! Being on a plant-based diet in a foreign country wasn't exactly easy! Albeit Subway wasn't the best choice in the world, but having simplicity and access to a vegan-friendly meal really kept my morale up that I wouldn't have to settle or starve.

Fast-forward to the UK a few weeks later. The holiday was lots of fun, and I was talking to someone about it. They asked me how the plant-based diet went over there, and I said it wasn't ideal, but finding Subway made it a bit easier, though not the best. After the conversation, I suddenly wondered, what exactly is in that veggie patty? I hadn't given it any thought before. But checking online, it bloody turned out to have cow's milk and eggs in it!

I didn't know back then, but there's a top-notch website called Happy Cow. It was founded in 1999 as a public service to help people find veggie/vegan options and healthy food. All you have to do is search the area you're in and voila! You get a list of places to eat, and how far they are from your location. All with links to prospective restaurants, bars, cafes, and health food stores. When going abroad, this website avoids any kind of Subway sitch! **happycow.net**

"You should be able to let your hair down and eat what you like on holiday"

A 2013 study found that 42% of people diet before going on holiday. And almost 80% gain weight while they're away. Plus, only 4% pay attention to the nutritional content of what they're eating on holiday. This shows how much people care about how they look when they go away, "the beach bod", but how little they care when they're home.

Another study pointed out that for some people, weight gained on holiday never comes off! Holidaying in the U.S. saw the highest weight gain over a 2-week period, at 8lb. The Caribbean, France, and Italy had just over a 7lb gain. Besides the enormous portions, all you can eat buffets, creamy sauces, and cheese common in these countries, the weight gain ultimately comes from being in a caloric surplus. Too much food and too little exercise.

If this is your idea of what a holiday is about, then you may be more susceptible to thinking that your vegan diet doesn't apply so much while you're away. Perhaps you're looking forward to a "guilt-free" holiday, where the guilt is free until you get home.

But you have to ask yourself: do you consider eating animals or animal products a treat? Do you consider it desirable? Do you want to work your arse off to pay for a holiday where you eat animals or animal products?

The standards you have towards your diet will ultimately dictate what you see as "letting your hair down" while you're on holiday. What's more, if you're looking for an escape from your diet, then it must be creating pressure and probably needs adjusting anyway.

Living with non-vegans

At the start of the plant-based transition, I was living at home with my mum and sister. In these earlier stages, I was prone to making fundamental mistakes. Sometimes, I'd make lots of effort to keep my diet up 24/7, without any regard for those I lived with, and therefore shared a fridge with!

If I had lived on my own, it would have been a different story. But going from one shelf per family member to suddenly taking over everyone's shelves for my food seemed wanky. My selfishness was making my vegan diet look bad, so I had to defend and justify it with factual evidence. Even so, my mum and sister questioned the necessity and rationale behind switching from a nutritional system that seemed to work well for me up to now. And the fridge system that worked so well for the household.

The situation couldn't go on for much longer, primarily because I didn't want to fall out with my family. But also because my diet had seemingly turned me into a selfish person. The kind of selfish person who takes over your fridge and then has a debate with you about it!

I attempted to do smaller food shops to take up less room in the fridge. This didn't impact my nutrition too much, because I planned my meals better in advance. It also meant less food waste. Trying to be too perfect with my nutrition meant buying so much food that it went off before I got round to prepping it. The sucky downside was finding time to go shopping more often.

The most important lesson I took from living with non-vegans is to keep unity in your household as best you can when making the transition to a plant-based diet. Whatever stage you're at. That or buy a second fridge!

Then I lived with my dad. I was more experienced in my diet, and I knew things would be a more easy-going with my dad—more banter. From the previous experience, I stuck to my designated areas in the kitchen. This meant me and my dad could focus on the funny side of our differences.

There were inevitably times when he questioned the necessity of the vegan thing and why I couldn't just have what he was having. But the same goes with the public. Call it "mainstream understanding of a plant-based diet". The difference is that your family will probably be more honest about their feelings. In which case, you have to be patient and empathetic—not get riled up, let it get to you, or feel attacked.

The most important lesson I took from the second experience was: the less you talk about being a vegan at home and the less serious you make it, the more fun you can have by giving it back to them!

"My parents won't let me take up a vegan diet"

Let's say you've got the vegan vibes. You hate eating meat, and feel shit inside and out. You'd rather not eat anything that comes from an animal because it doesn't feel right. And you've researched the knock-on the effects of the diet. So you know why you feel this way.

What are you waiting for? You're made for this diet! But then, oh wait. Your family don't approve. They hate vegan stuff. They've basically banned you because they think it's for bloody hippies. You don't want to alienate yourself from your family or for them to be ashamed of you. So what do you do?

It all depends on your situation. Do you live at home? Are you old enough to look after yourself and make your own decisions? What type of relationship do you have with your parents? Can you be open with them? Have you had conversations with them about trying a vegan diet before? How did they take it? What's the worst that could happen? Would they disown you?

Taking everything into account, my advice is to not make a big deal out of it. Judge the situation first. Before you mention anything, do you even have to use the "V word"? If the vegan thing is what they oppose, then maybe you can just say you're going to cut out meat, fish, and animal products. You can even do it gradually to avoid suspicion if you really feel you can't be honest.

Personally, when first mentioning my diet change to my family, I didn't avoid the "V word". And they did freak a little. But they also said "As long as you know what you're doing and have done your research, we're happy" etc. Their main concern was that I'd lose all the muscle I had worked so hard for, and that there was no need to change because everything seemed good as it was. Their apprehensions were just like mine initially. So I explained I would take it slowly and experiment, which appealed to them!

If your family are okay with you trying the diet but they buy all the food at home, then you may not have control over what goes in your home. But you still have control over what goes in your stomach. Likewise if you live with your friends or partner. Just try to avoid clashing with those at home over your diet. At dinner times where everyone is eating together, you could provide your own foods. Or just don't eat the non-vegan-friendly ingredients.

Whatever the case, stay open to their objections. Listen more, so you can respond better. Show empathy and appreciation for their concerns. Let your actions do the talking by keeping yourself fit and healthy, and not taking over the fridge. Let the vegan conversation come to you, and direct your family to any references you feel will help them understand your position.

The elephant in the room

When people talk about feeling tired, sick, weak, stressed, fat, and so on, the solution to their problems isn't rocket science. It's often dietary and exercise-related, and could be improved if they had a healthier lifestyle. More often than not, people already know what the root cause of their problems is. Too much junk food and not enough fruit and vegetables.

When people spoke to me about their diet or health, having listened to their understanding of why they feel rubbish, I could more or less guarantee that they weren't getting enough micronutrients. Plain and simple. The calories were there, but the nutrients weren't. In these cases, I would prescribe the classic "sounds like you need to eat more fruits and vegetables, and less processed foods, including animal products" in the least patronising way.

If the conversation got deeper, I might suggest a "plant-based diet" instead of the words "vegan diet". It's like the PG-rated version– it doesn't offend! I also didn't want to debate why they couldn't reduce their animal product consumption for personal reasons such as enjoyment, habit, convenience, etc.

So, I used it in the context of "the easiest way to focus on getting more fruits and vegetables in your diet is to eat a plant-based diet". Or, if I was trying to avoid a debate, a "mostly plant-based diet".

The elephant in the room was the benefits of a plant-based diet, and it wasn't just present in conversations about general lifestyle either. It would also come up in conversations about cholesterol. For example, if someone got a raised or high cholesterol reading, they would take it as a specific problem area that was letting their health down overall, not an overall problem.

Usually, their doctor had prescribed controlling their cholesterol through diet. They would tell me they'd tried certain food habits to reduce it, such as eating more monounsaturated fats in avocados, nuts, and seeds to improve 'good' cholesterol. But to no avail–their cholesterol was still on the rise.

Then I would find out they were still eating animal products with these foods. So I'd discuss the potential link between animal products and cholesterol, even letting them know that my cholesterol had gone from an "okay" reading to "low" since adopting a plant-based diet. But I was met with the same reasons for not wanting to reduce or abstain from animal products.

Eventually, it turned out that the only thing they hadn't tried in order to reduce their cholesterol was to reduce or abstain from their animal product consumption. Yet it still wasn't worth trying to them, even when they said they'd always struggled with their cholesterol. I don't know about you, but if I had an issue with my cholesterol never going down when I'd tried other things, I'd be giving any other advice a go. Especially if nothing else seemed to be working.

The whole thing reminded me of the true definition of detox, which we looked at before. Often, the answer may not be eating other foods on top of the foods you're already eating. The answer may be in abstaining from foods that you're already eating

"The vegan diet has to be done a certain way"

The most popular diet in the UK as of 2014 was a calorie restriction for five days a week, then unconstrained eating for two days a week, commonly called the 5-2 diet. A reported 39% of diet followers chose this option. Low-carb, high-fat diets came in second, with 32% of diet followers choosing it. High-protein, low-fat plans were third, with 25% of the vote.

The only criteria of a plant-based diet is to not eat foods that contain animal products. Other than that, you can basically do whatever you want with your diet. There are no calorie restrictions, set food timings, or set ingredients, etc.

If you were to think beyond the diet and look at other lifestyle elements, the general criteria of a vegan lifestyle is to not use animal products. So, you'd need to take more due diligence in buying health and beauty products, clothing, accessories, etc.

Unless you've been living under a rock, then you'll know that for many of these products to exist, animals have been affected. Not just directly through inflicted pain and suffering in being tested on, but indirectly as their habitats are destroyed in the process, causing grief and contributing to extinction.

Think about all the arguments and reasons we've covered up to now for wanting to adopt a plant-based diet. Ethics, the environment, health, cost, etc. But how about just because of logic?

Logic is defined as: reasoning conducted or assessed according to strict principals of validity. In this case, logic is brought about through a combination of intuition, experience, and research. When I realised the bigger, positive impact on everything associated with the vegan diet, it appealed to me massively. Logic told me that the alternative wasn't right.

So, as well as looking for animal products in my food, I try to do the same for health and beauty products, clothing, and accessories. To the best of my due diligence and knowledge at the time, I try not to use anything that has been tested on animals, because the thought and sight of it, having looked into it, is fucking disgraceful.

The biggest impact and difference you can ever make to animals, to the environment, to your health, and society doesn't always have to be come via a loud protest. You can vote for, look out for, and support all of these things with your pound, dollar, or whatever currency you use.

The more you purchase animal products, be it food or things that have been tested on animals, the greater the demand. In business terms, this means the greater the supply. This means more suffering. If you stop purchasing these items, the lower the demand. Meaning lower the supply, lower the suffering.

The other side is that companies look to supply for this new demand. The demand for vegan food, vegan-friendly products, and cruelty-free products, plus advances in technology will bring a more extensive range and quantity of vegan-friendly products. It will also bring a less extensive range and quantity of non-vegan friendly products. Your demand, alongside others who share the same vote, will bring less suffering and will subsequently change the mainstream to include less animal products.

If you follow the vegan diet, it isn't done a certain way. It's done your way. Your way will be based on what you feel you need to do. And how far you feel you need to go. And it will purely be based on what you consider to be logical action based on your intuition, experience, and research.

If you need to go beyond the diet to do this, if you want to adopt the lifestyle, then that's your way!

VEGAN summary

You are what you say you are.

If you go around telling everyone that you're a "vegan", then you will be known as "(insert your name) the vegan" to others. Strategically decide how you want to make your nutritional requirements known to others in society.

Eat more fruit than ever before.

Presumably, you eat around five portions a day or less, going by the UK averages. Increase this by incorporating fruit at meal times as dessert, and in between meals as snacks. You can also integrate more fruit juice or smoothies (not from concentrate).

Identify whether you really need supplements before taking them.

Before buying any supplement, ask yourself, "Do I really need this?" And "What is it going to do for me?" If you genuinely can't answer these questions, then maybe you just need to pick your nutrition more wisely to suit your goals.

Always train and eat to your goals.

Taking part in any form of exercise will have its benefits. But training and eating to your goals is another thing. Make sure you know what you want to achieve before starting a protocol with either. That way, you'll be happier when you progress.

Use Cronometer to track your macro and micronutrient intake.

MyFitnessPal only shows your micronutrient intake to a very basic degree. Cronometer covers micronutrients in more depth and can make you more aware of any potential deficiencies in your current diet.

BBQs are for everyone to enjoy.

At BBQs always take your own food and provide something that everyone can enjoy. This way, you stay involved with your friends as normal and won't stand out as being difficult to cater for.

Never start a debate with someone about plant-based diets.

Understand that you are not the spokesperson for all vegans and you only represent you in your own words and actions. If you do start a debate, it's likely to be met with frustration and aggression from the other side. Either online or in person. It's pointless.

Holidays are for everyone to enjoy.

Be as practical as you possibly can when on holiday. Granted, it's not always the most ideal situation. But do what you can to keep to your diet if you want to come back "guilt-free".

Try not to shit too much where you eat.

Drawing attention to yourself in your household by not conforming to your previous standards of etiquette won't gain you many fans at home. Even though your diet is changing, it doesn't mean that your values should.

People already know about the elephant in the room.

A plant-based diet has been about for centuries. Specific studies relating to its benefits can be found across the internet and in books. Everyone knows it's there. But do they look for it? No. Do they care about it? Maybe not.

It isn't as much of a big deal as people think.

There may come a time where you barely have to think about anything vegan-related. You just function on autopilot and it all seems completely normal to you. If anything, you might wonder what all the noise is about!

WHAT NOW?

Noteworthy things to take your knowledge further

Documentaries

My favourite documentaries to watch early on were mostly available on Netflix. Some are undoubtedly better than others, but each gives little gold nuggets of information that I could take on board and digest easily.

Individually, they helped me understand specific aspects related to the diet and lifestyle, such as implications on health, the environment, society, and ethics. Collectively, they helped me understand everything better (cringe alert)!

Because of these factors, I'm happy to recommend these documentaries (in no particular order):

- Earthlings.
- What the Health.
- Food, Inc.
- Cowspiracy: The Sustainability Secret.
- GMO OMG.
- Forks Over Knives.
- Rotten.
- Food Matters.
- Blackfish.
- Fat, Sick & Nearly Dead.
- Engine 2 Diet.
- Vegucated.

The information provided in these documentaries is often referenced, with appearances and insights from some of the most well-known people in the relevant industries.

YouTube

When it comes to YouTube, you have no idea if what you type in will provide you with a good, credible video or not! Some of the most popular ones aren't the best sources of information—they're just entertaining. I guess you could say the cream doesn't always rise to the top on YouTube, and you'll definitely have to kiss a few frogs before you find what you're looking for.

Even so, it's nice to get another perspective on the diet and vegan stuff. Whether they're knowledgeable and credible or purely entertaining, I recommend typing in any queries you have and seeing what you get back.

Follow on social media

From the documentaries and good YouTube channels, you have the opportunity to take your new-found knowledge further by "following" the featured spokespeople so you can keep tabs on their work and their perspective on research. I highly recommend following Dr Michael Greger and looking into his website: **nutritionfacts.org**. They also have an informative Youtube channel. Even for meat-eaters or non-vegans, the information provided on all things nutrition and health could be useful.

Other than my above recommendation, I'm not going to coerce you into following someone just because I related to them at the time of writing this. So I'll let you be the judge of who you follow based on whether you like them and can relate to them. It's a lot easier to build your list of credible people to follow than you'd think. Every time you add someone on social media these days, you get a pop-up with suggestions. This will take you from one reputable and credible person to the next.

Unfollow on social media

I also did a lot of "unfollowing". If I wanted to concentrate on and retain as much new information as possible, I had to get ruthless and clear out some old stuff to make room. The first things I unfollowed on social media were ego-driven pages and people: any salesy, supplementy, selfie, ranty, moany, or political stuff. It's embarrassing that half the stuff was on my page in the first place. So it was actually quite therapeutic to unfollow them.

Books

You'll find that many of the credible people you come across in the documentaries have their own books on their specialist subject.

I personally digest information better through other means, so I tend to watch documentaries and listen to podcasts more than read. You may be a bookworm, so go with what interests and who you warm to in the documentaries.

Podcasts

Of all the sources, this is my most utilised. Reason being, you can multitask and be active while you listen. You can be driving, walking, running, cycling, basically getting on with life, all while information and research trickles into your ears and hopefully into your brain!

You may find that your favourite spokespeople on social media, YouTube, or documentaries have their own podcast. Or have appeared as guests on other people's podcasts. Collaboration of hosts is very common across podcasts channels. You'll learn so much from being a fly on the wall eavesdropping. I recommend starting with The Rich Roll Podcast and going from there. He's a ledge and has interesting guests who are often clued up on fitness, health and nutrition.

Listening more

Listening more is how I heard the majority of the misconceptions in this book, beyond my own initial concerns about the diet. In fact, the best part of following up on these anecdotes was that I had subjectively believed some of them to be true prior to looking into them objectively.

I'd mentally note what people said, and sometimes put it in a reminders list. Then I'd check whether there was any truth in it. Nothing fancy was needed to find the answers—just some credible, unbiased websites. If you do this yourself, you may find that you learn more than the original subject you were looking into, as it's easy to go off on a tangent!

"What made you go vegan?"

Of all the questions I've been asked since making the final stage, this one has to be the most popular. I get asked this question around once a week. It's weird because I sometimes get it from people I haven't known all that long, and sometimes from older friends and acquaintances who just haven't asked me before.

Truth be told, I have no idea what the original answer to this question was! Nowadays, I know it's because of logic. But looking back, there wasn't a particular thing, a breaking point as such. As you've seen from reading my story, there was definitely a series of events that seemed to accumulate in a short space of time.

At one point, I remember thinking that I was being bombarded and overwhelmed with one sign after the other to go vegan! But I didn't go vegan overnight; it was gradual. From one stage to the next.

Because of this, I find it very difficult to give a specific answer. I wouldn't want to give someone my life story and go through every single event that led to this point. Ain't nobody got time for that! Plus, I wouldn't want to make it out to be a big deal. To make ends meet, I avoid specifics and go with a blanket answer of: "I just felt like I wanted to do it, so I looked into it for a while before trying it and here we are!"

I have found that the less you say, and the more general your answer, the less you will need to say. If your response is too long or specific, for example, "Oh, I did it for the animals because of X, Y, and Z", this can lead to tangents and other questions. It could lead to them getting confused (and potentially irate), which means more questions for you!

My general answer always seems to be followed up with, "So did you do it overnight or did you phase everything out gradually?" To which I say "gradually" and the conversation goes from there.

As I'm generally around 'fitnessy' people, the kind of questions I get asked are about protein intake, muscle loss, carbs making you fat, or supplements. My answer is again short and sweet. If there is more debate from there, I very subtly state that "I've done my research, I know how I feel, and I like it."

If you need any guidance on how you could answer questions better, you can refer back to the misconceptions. To save time explaining, you could even recommend that they read this book!

When you hear an outsider's perspective on a plant-based diet, eating only vegan-friendly food seems to be the hardest thing about the diet. However, perhaps the most difficult part, at least in the beginning, is the planning and information side of it all.

It involves knowing what food you need to buy, the nutrients it will provide, reading this book and perhaps others, listening to podcasts, setting up apps such as Cronometer to get your micronutrient requirements, buying the right food in the right amounts, using Happy Cow, and so on. You may feel like you're learning this stuff from scratch. Like it's an uphill battle. But once you've done the research prior to buying the food, eating it is the easy and fun part!

Hopefully, if you put in the initial effort to get an understanding and enough confidence to get you going, you'll learn the rest along the way. Yes, through getting your hands dirty and making a few mistakes! The good thing is that in times like these, you will literally Think and Grow Vegan for the next time, so you won't make the same mistake twice.

Now for the motivational spiel... You may have acquired this book to help you on your journey. However, buying it alone won't guarantee you success with this. Neither will just reading it. If you wish to make the most of the content, you should apply whatever information best resonates with you and your lifestyle, wherever suitable.

In other words, if you've got to this stage of the book, and you still haven't attempted a plant-based diet but you want to try it, or you tried and gave up but you still want to try again, then as mentioned in the very beginning; fucking go for it!

Disclaimer

Glen John Jones is not in connection with any medical facility neither is he a medical professional. The information provided in this book should not be used as a substitute for the counsel of an experienced medical professional. Many people have made successful progress through using Glen John Jones's services or products. There are, however, many factors that impact whether an individual person will make successful progress. Any service or product provided by Glen John Jones has its limitations, and he can make no guarantees about its effectiveness for every individual.

The information contained in this book is Glen John Jones's opinions based on research and personal experience unless otherwise stated, and should not be substituted for qualified medical advice. Health related information is in no way intended to diagnose, prevent, treat or cure any medical or other condition. Always seek the counsel of a qualified medical practitioner or other health care provider for an individual consultation before making any significant changes to your nutrition and/or lifestyle. This includes prior to starting any training/nutritional program designed by Glen John Jones and prior to implementing any service or product provided by Glen John Jones.

Any links to external web sites are provided as a courtesy only. Glen John Jones does not endorse the content or views expressed by any third parties (including post and page comments) unless otherwise stated. It is the responsibility of each individual user to determine the accuracy and personal relevance of any information found in this book or in any linked materials. Glen John Jones assumes no responsibility or liability for any consequences resulting directly or indirectly from any action or inaction taken as a result of following information contained in this book or in any linked materials. This includes any training/nutritional programme designed by Glen John Jones or any service or product provided by Glen John Jones.

Thanks for reading!

This subject can often bring about more questions
to the answers you find along the way!

For any further information, future publications
or if you have any queries relating to your own
plant-based diet please visit: **thinkandgrowvegan.com**

I'd also love to hear more about what
you thought of this book. Please leave a review.